Selective Antibiotic Use in Respiratory Illness
A Family Practice Guide

Dedicated to

Iris
Karen, John and Adrian

Selective Antibiotic Use in Respiratory Illness: a Family Practice Guide

M. T. Everett MB, BS, FRCS
General Practitioner, Plymouth

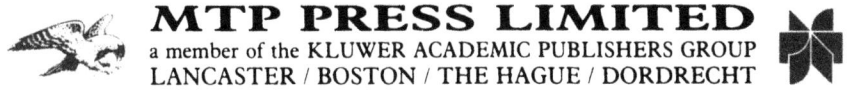

MTP PRESS LIMITED
a member of the KLUWER ACADEMIC PUBLISHERS GROUP
LANCASTER / BOSTON / THE HAGUE / DORDRECHT

Erratum:

P 123. In the section on Bronchodilators and Steroids the dose for prednisolone should have been given as 10mg immediately, followed by 5 mg 3 times a day.

Published in the UK and Europe by
MTP Press Limited
Falcon House
Lancaster, England

British Library Cataloguing in Publication Data

Everett, M. T.
  Selective antibiotic use in respiratory
  illness: a family practice guide,
  1. Respiratory organs—Diseases—
  Chemotherapy   2. Antibiotics
  I. Title
  615'.72   RC735.A57

  ISBN 978-94-015-1145-2   ISBN 978-94-015-1143-8 (eBook)
  DOI 10.1007/978-94-015-1143-8

Published in the USA by
MTP Press
A division of Kluwer Boston Inc
190 Old Derby Street
Hingham, MA 02043, USA

Copyright © 1986 MTP Press Ltd
Softcover reprint of the hardcover 1st edition 1986

All rights reserved. No part of this publication may be reproduced, stored in a retrieval system, or transmitted in any form or by any means, electronic, mechanical, photocopying, recording or otherwise, without prior permission from the publishers.

Phototypesetting by Georgia Origination, Liverpool.

Contents

Preface   vii

Acknowledgements   viii

1 Antibiotics and the Patient   1
Allergy – Antibiotic Diarrhoea – The Contraceptive Pill – Pregnancy – Lactation – Neonates – Children – The Elderly – Hepatic and Renal Impairment – Drug Interactions – Absorption

2 Management Principles   21

3 Pyrexia   31
Febrile Convulsions – Delirium – Rigors – Symptomatic Management of Pyrexia – Antibiotic Use

4 Sore Throat, Tonsillitis and Pharyngitis   41
Definition – The Non-inflamed Sore Throat – The Inflamed Throat – Referral for Tonsillectomy

5 Otitis Media   65
Use of the Auroscope – Clinical Features of Acute Otitis Media – Bacteria in Acute Otitis Media – Secretory Otitis Media – Management and Antibiotic Use – Chronic Otitis Media

Selective Antibiotic Use in Respiratory Illness

6 Sinusitis — 83
Clinical Features – Bacteriology – Management and Antibiotic Use

7 Laryngitis — 91
Croup – Hoarseness or Loss of Voice

8 Coughs and Colds — 99
The Acute Cough – Cold in the Nose – Persistent Cough in Children – Persistent Cough in Adults – The Absent Cough

9 Wheezy Bronchitis in Children — 121
The Nature of Wheezy Bronchitis – Recognition of Asthma – Management of the Acute Episode – Longer-term Management – Differential Diagnosis

10 Pneumonia — 135
Clinical Diagnosis – Investigation – Infective Causes – Management and Antibiotic Use – Differential Diagnosis

11 Bronchitis, Bronchiolitis and Bronchiectasis — 159
Acute Bronchitis – Acute Bronchiolitis – Chronic Bronchitis – Bronchiectasis

12 Vomiting and Diarrhoea — 169
Non-specific Vomiting – Gastro-enteritis – Management

13 PUO in Children — 181
Definition – Emergent Diagnoses – Management and Antibiotic Use

14 Influenza and the 'Flu-like Illness — 189
The Influenzal Illness – Viral Causes – Differential Diagnosis – Clinical Assessment of the Patient with 'Flu – Management and Antibiotic Use

Index — 205

Preface

The purpose of this book is to clarify the use of antibiotics in the management of the common respiratory illnesses seen in general practice. The underlying philosophy, which embraces the avoidance of unnecessary use, is that proper use entails a full understanding of the nature of the illness.

The concept of selective antibiotic use recognizes that respiratory illnesses commonly comprise multiple illness features, and that some of these features have a viral cause and some a bacterial one. In assessing antibiotic need, each feature or component part of an illness may be evaluated individually, so enabling a decision for antibiotic use in the illness as a whole.

The nature of each individual illness feature with its antibiotic indication is discussed in successive chapters, and this accumulated knowledge is of value in managing the more complex PUO and flu-like illnesses which are discussed at the end of the book.

The first two chapters encompass the principles of antibiotic use and the relationship between antibiotic prescribing and various states of the patient, e.g. allergy, pregnancy etc.

An attempt has been made to justify every recommendation or decision, and non-antibiotic management is discussed where relevant.

Acknowledgements

I acknowledge a long association with the Plymouth Public Health Laboratory, and am indebted to Dr P. D. Meers, past Director; Dr P. J. Wilkinson, Director; Dr G. M. Churcher, Consultant Microbiologist and Cytopathologist, and Dr S. Reilly, Consultant Microbiologist. I also acknowledge the contribution made by the Domiciliary X-ray service, and am indebted to the late Dr E. A. Waldron; Dr W. H. Smith, Dr P. F. Norman, and Dr R. M. Paxton, Consultant Radiologists.

I wish to express my thanks to Miss V. M. Trinder and Mrs J. Elliott of the Plymouth Medical Library for the trouble they took in obtaining photostats of numerous papers. I also wish to thank Professor D. F. Hawkins of the Institute of Obstetrics and Gynaecology, The Hammersmith Hospital, for access to his manuscript on antibiotics and pregnancy long before its publication, and Professor D. Vere of the Department of Pharmacology and Therapeutics, The London Hospital Medical College, for correspondence relating to the absorption of anticonvulsant drugs. I acknowledge the contribution made by two past Editors of the *Journal of the Royal College of General Practitioners*, Dr D. J. Pereira Gray and Dr S. L. Barley, in stimulating thought.

I am grateful to Searle & Co. Ltd. for information relating to interaction between antibiotics and progesterone-only pills. A colleague and her son very kindly sat for the photographs in Chapter 5. Miss Sue Payne of Tavistock typed both the original and final manuscripts with great skill and accuracy.

1
Antibiotics and the Patient

Allergy – Antibiotic Diarrhoea – The Contraceptive Pill – Pregnancy – Lactation – Neonates – Children – The Elderly – Hepatic and Renal Impairment – Drug Interactions – Absorption

The use of any drug entails more than a consideration of the disease itself. When prescribing an antibiotic, the possibility of inducing an allergic reaction and of inducing antibiotic diarrhoea is borne in mind, and of the many states of the patient, the possibility of pregnancy is never far from the general practitioner's thoughts.

ALLERGY

Allergy to Penicillin

Allergic reactions are caused more commonly by penicillin than by other antibiotics, and a story of allergy to one type of penicillin must be assumed to reflect allergy to all types. This is because all penicillins contain the 6-aminopenicillanic acid nucleus from which the responsible major and minor determinants are derived. Enquiry of known allergy should be made when the use of penicillin is proposed, and this serves to prevent some reactions, but many instances of allergy occur despite previous safe use.

Anaphylactic Shock

This, the most severe reaction, develops between three and 30 minutes after dosage and may be fatal. This type of reaction is rare and has occurred usually after parenteral dosage, but instances following the use of oral penicillin are described (Simmonds *et al.* 1978, Schwartz and Sher 1984). If a general practitioner has had the experience of a patient 'collapsing on the end of the needle', he will probably never give intramuscular penicillin again; fortunately patients needing antibiotics in general practice can invariably be managed using the oral route.

The clinical features of anaphylactic shock comprise hypotension, tachycardia, loss of consciousness, and in addition, there may be other allergic features, e.g. laryngeal oedema or asthma, and the patient may become severely cyanosed.

Emergency treatment comprises intra-muscular adrenaline (0.5 ml of 1 in 1000) which may need to be repeated at quarter-hourly intervals, and intravenous hydrocortisone in a dose of 100 or 200 mg, and intravenous chlorpheniramine in a dose of 10 or 20 mg. The establishment of an artificial airway may be necessary, e.g. a large-bore needle through the cricothyroid membrane or a laryngotomy, again through the cricothyroid membrane (Chapter 7).

Other Allergic Reactions

Cutaneous urticaria is unquestionably an allergic reaction and can be managed by oral antihistamines, but the urticaria may involve the mouth and pharynx, and sometimes the larynx, when a life-threatening situation develops. Management then follows the same lines as for anaphylactic shock. Severe asthma will also be helped by intravenous hydrocortisone, but now, nebulized salbutamol would be used as well.

The most common allergic reaction is the maculo-papular rash which can develop up to several days after antibiotic use. There is no life-threatening situation, and the use of oral antihistamines plus stopping the penicillin is adequate management. The problem is that many such instances may not represent allergy but reflect the illness itself. This dilemma invariably occurs in children, and the diagnostic difficulties can be caused by rubella, modified measles (i.e. modified by immunization) and the less well-known enterovirus rashes. Although a typical exanthem progresses from the neck downwards while an allergic rash appears everywhere at once, the distinction in clinical practice is often difficult.

Ampicillin Allergy in Glandular Fever

It is now well-known that the common maculo-papular rash following the use of ampicillin in a patient with glandular fever does not usually represent allergy. The same phenomenon can occur in patients with leukaemia, cytomegalovirus infection, and in those with a high serum uric acid. The same phenomenon can also be caused by amoxycillin and by augmentin (clavulanate-potentiated amoxycillin).

The problem facing the doctor is whether it is safe to use the penicillins subsequently. If the reaction was urticarial, then the penicillins should certainly not be used again. If the reaction was maculo-papular, then their subsequent use probably will be safe but in fact, for the sake of certainty, an alternative antibiotic usually will be used. The dilemma can be prevented by avoiding the use of ampicillin or amoxycillin (or augmentin) in patients with glandular fever or if glandular fever is suspected.

Cross-reaction with Cephalosporins

The clinical incidence of cross allergy to the cephalosporins in patients known to be allergic to penicillin varies between 5 and 9% (Dash 1975, Petz 1978), and wheal-and-flare skin tests with cephalothin were unequivocally positive in 49% of 74 subjects who were allergic to penicillin (Sullivan 1984). The type of allergic reaction is not confined to the skin; both fatal and non-fatal anaphylaxis have been recorded.

If the history of penicillin allergy includes urticaria, angio-oedema, asthma, laryngeal oedema, or hypotension, a cephalosporin should certainly not be given. The risk of cross-reactivity is less likely if the history of penicillin allergy is represented only by a skin rash, but certainty can be established only by skin testing, and in the home management of patients an alternative to both penicillin and cephalosporin should be used.

Skin Testing and Desensitization

Once applied, the penicillin-allergic label tends to adhere for life, and this can present treatment problems often years later, e.g. during pregnancy, or if a particular bacterium is resistant to certain antibiotics, or if a particular antibiotic is known to cause diarrhoea. Inevitably, therefore, thought has been given to whether the penicillins or cephalosporins could be used again despite the label. The following considerations are relevant to this concept.

(1) *The patient may not be allergic to penicillin* The allergy label is most often applied during childhood and most often following a rash, but the rash will sometimes be caused by the illness itself, and Madden (1977) emphasizes the importance of detail in labelling. Re-exposure to penicillin caused a reaction in only four of 28 adults (Oswald 1983), and allergy is also known to wane with time (Patterson and Anderson 1982).

(2) *Skin tests and desensitization* For skin testing to be reliable, it is necessary to test against the whole battery of major and minor penicillin determinants; penicilloyl poly-L-lysine, penicillin G and penicilloic acid. Although it has been suggested that skin testing might be carried out in the surgery with proper safeguards (Madden 1977), most doctors would feel the tests should be undertaken in a hospital department where the patient is better placed should a rare serious reaction occur.

Desensitization by injection has tended to be little used owing to the possible hazard and because several days are needed to encompass the increasing doses, but Sullivan *et al.* (1982) have achieved both speed and safety by *oral* desensitization.

Polio Immunization

Oral poliomyelitis vaccine contains trace amounts of penicillin which were present in the original seed strain and cannot be bred out. Of relevance to the general practitioner is the safety of giving polio vaccine in the presence of believed penicillin allergy. The dilemma is fed by the knowledge that, very rarely, trace amounts of penicillin, even administered orally, can be the cause of anaphylaxis (Schwartz and Sher 1984).

The clinical situation is usually a small child who may already have had one or two staged immunizations, but has now been labelled allergic to penicillin. Should the third dose be given? Should the pre-school booster later on be given? Should polio vaccine be given later in adult life for foreign travel?

The strict answer is no, but it is known that many of the alleged allergic rashes in small children reflect the illness itself. In practical terms, if the allergic reaction was represented by urticaria, asthma, laryngeal oedema or anaphylactic shock, then polio vaccine should not be given on any subsequent occasion. If, however, the reaction was a maculopapular rash, then the risk is extremely small. The risk, however, is not absent, and the decision ultimately rests between the patient and the practitioner concerned.

Allergy to Other Antibiotics

Other commonly used antimicrobial drugs present less of a problem. Sulphonamides may sometimes cause an allergic rash, which, when occurring after the use of cotrimoxazole, is attributed to its sulphamethoxazole component. Allergic reactions to trimethoprim do occur but are uncommon, and allergic reactions to erythromycin and to the tetracyclines have been described but rarely occur.

Prevention of Allergy

Question of allergy should be made prior to the use of an antibiotic, and will serve to prevent some occurrences, but more significantly, an attempt can be made to reduce the incidence of allergy to penicillin occurring in the first place. The single most useful method is to avoid unnecessary antibiotic use (Chapter 2). Refinements in antibiotic choice can also help. Grob (1977) has suggested the use of erythromycin as a first choice for the treatment of tonsillitis (Chapter 4), and prudent antibiotic choice may prevent confusion between exanthem and allergy. If a child, for example, is suspected of being in the prodromal phase of measles and needs an antibiotic, then the choice of an antibiotic other than penicillin will reduce confusion should a rash develop.

ANTIBIOTIC DIARRHOEA

Of antibiotics in common usage in general practice, diarrhoea is most often caused by ampicillin, and less often by amoxycillin and erythromycin. The cephalosporins and co-trimoxazole are usually free from this side effect. The tetracyclines rarely seem to cause diarrhoea, but this impression may be due to their less frequent use, i.e. avoidance in childhood.

It is a common experience that patients given an antibiotic who develop loose stools will almost invariably do so again if given the same antibiotic on a subsequent occasion. The explanation is probably not superinfection but a mucosal toxic effect (*British Medical Journal* 1975).

Management and Prevention

Antibiotic diarrhoea is nearly always non-serious, and it is sufficient to stop the antibiotic and the diarrhoea will invariably cease within 24 hours. Attempts at prevention, however, are worthwhile, because the presence of diarrhoea is inconvenient and carries the rare risk of pseudomembranous colitis. Just as in preventing allergic reactions, the avoidance of unnecessary use and the prudent choice of antibiotic can minimize the problem. Question of previous diarrhoea may enable avoidance of the same antibiotic again. If an illness needs an antibiotic and is exhibiting diarrhoea as part of that illness, or if the patient has a colostomy or ileostomy, then an antibiotic without diarrhoea potential is preferable.

Pseudomembranous Colitis

Pseudomembranous colitis is very uncommon and will rarely if ever be seen by an individual general practitioner. The disorder can be associated with almost any antibiotic, but most instances have occurred after the use of lincomycin or clindamycin. These two antibiotics are now seldom used, and the antibiotic management of patients in general practice is possible without recourse to their use at all.

The cause is nearly always the cytopathic toxin of *Clostridium difficile*, and only rarely is a staphylococcal overgrowth responsible. The clinical features comprise profuse and possibly blood-stained diarrhoea, colicky abdominal pain, nausea, weakness, tachycardia, fever and abdominal distension. Electrolyte imbalance and loss of albumen into the gut occur, and the more severe illnesses can result in megacolon, perforation, peritonitis and death. Diagnosis is made by sigmoidoscopy when the pseudomembrane is seen, and biopsy taken. Treatment entails supportive measures in hospital, and the specific use of vancomycin given orally in a dose of 125–500 mg six hourly for 5–10 days. Metronidazole is an effective alternative (Teasley *et al.* 1983).

THE CONTRACEPTIVE PILL

In common with phenobarbitone, phenytoin, primidone, and carbamezapine, antibiotics can also impair the efficacy of the pill.

The Combined Pill

The risk of an unwanted pregnancy is quite high among women taking rifampicin (Reimers *et al.* 1974), and although the risk with other antibiotics is much lower, a wide spectrum of antibiotics have been implicated including the penicillins, tetracyclines, co-trimoxazole, cephalosporins, and metronidazole (Dossetor 1975, Stockley 1982, Fraser and Jansen 1983).

Management

In practice, one rare and two common clinical situations are met.

(1) A general practitioner rarely will have a patient in the practice on long-term rifampicin for tuberculosis. A corollary may be drawn with those on anticonvulsants for epilepsy, when the use of a high dose pill of 50 μg or 80 μg (50 μg plus 30 μg) is believed to prevent the adverse interaction between anticonvulsant and pill, but the relatively long-term use of a pill of this strength is possibly unacceptable, and the better advice is to recommend an alternative method of contraception. The progesterone-only pill is acceptable because so far, there appear to be no reports of failure induced by rifampicin with progesterone-only pills (Stockley 1982).

(2) Tetracycline is commonly used on a long-term basis for the treatment of acne, and theoretically poses the additional risk of fetal abnormality should an unwanted pregnancy occur, but in fact the use of tetracycline is less of a problem than might seem apparent. The risk of fetal abnormality is probably smaller than believed (see section on pregnancy), and the incidence of unwanted pregnancy induced by interaction between tetracycline and the pill is very low – so low in fact, that use of the pill is probably preferable to less reliable and less acceptable methods of contraception, e.g. barrier methods.

Cunliffe (1984) reported no unwanted pregnancies among 525 sexually active patients treated for acne with six months tetracycline or erythromycin, and who used a 30 μg pill. If the patient had been using a 20 μg pill, then a change was made to 30 μg, and the patient advised to take extra precautions if diarrhoea occurred. These results are very reassuring but there is the exception. An unwanted pregnancy (Bacon and Shenfield 1980) occurred in a woman taking a 30 μg pill and given a five day course of tetracycline for sinusitis.

If the rare combined risks of tetracycline are to be totally eliminated, the option exists to treat acne with an alternative antibiotic, e.g. erythromycin.

(3) The most common situation is the patient who is given a short antibiotic course for chest, throat, sinus or ear. The strength of the pill cannot be altered in the context of a short antibiotic course, and the only possible advice is to take extra contraceptive precautions until the end of the packet.

The Progesterone-only Pill

Unpublished data (Searle and Co. Ltd. 1984) indicate one unwanted pregnancy attributed to the concurrent use of co-trimoxazole and a mini-pill, but there seem to be no other recorded instances. This apparent absence of adverse interaction is not unexpected because the progesterone-only pill exerts its contraceptive effect more by peripheral than central action.

PREGNANCY

The Mother

Owing to increased renal function in pregnancy, antibiotics have a 30–50% lower plasma level and a significantly shorter half-life than occurring in non-pregnant women (Philipson 1983). When treating maternal infections, therefore, the commonly used antibiotics may need to be given in a larger dose, particularly, for example, if the response is less than expected.

The Fetus

The knowledge that drugs cross the placenta can be used for the benefit of the fetus, but the greater concern, when prescribing drugs in pregnancy, is the avoidance of fetal abnormality. The doctor is obviously alert to this possibility when the patient is known to be pregnant, but the same care in prescribing relates to the whole child-bearing age because a patient might unknowingly be in very early pregnancy, or might conceive while taking the drug.

An accurate assessment of the safety of a drug is difficult; there is seldom proof of cause and effect. A fetal abnormality, for example, may have been caused by the disorder for which the drug was given, rather than by the drug itself. Sources of information on the safety of drug use in pregnancy include large surveys, partly controlled studies, serendipity, case reports, theoretical speculations, animal studies, and reviews (Hawkins 1985), and there are problems of interpretation related to each source. A full evaluation of these sources and of the mechanisms of teratogenesis led Hawkins (1985) to suggest that the risks of antibiotic use in pregnancy are less than generally believed.

The Penicillins, The Cephalosporins, Erythromycin and Metronidazole

Hawkins (1985) concluded that these four antibiotics (and local nystatin) are apparently harmless to the fetus at all stages of pregnancy. This conclusion is based upon several works including the large studies by Nelson and Forfar (1971) and by the Birmingham Research Unit of the Royal College of General Practitioners (1975).

The Penicillins

The conclusion of safety relates to the commonly used penicillins but not to the more recently available clavulanate-potentiated amoxycillin (augmentin). The safety of clavulanic acid in human pregnancy has yet to be established.

Metronidazole

American concern about the teratogenicity and mutagenicity of metronidazole in animals has caused their recommendation to avoid its use in the first trimester, but this advice seems groundless. Metronidazole was used for the treatment of Trichomonas infection in 597 of 880 patients so infected, out of a total of 9629 deliveries at the Hammersmith Hospital between 1971 and 1976 (Morgan 1978). A dose of 200 mg thrice daily for 7-10 days was received by 62 patients in the first trimester, 284 in the second and 251 in the third. The incidence of low birth weight infants, stillbirths and congenital abnormalities was unaffected by metronidazole treatment.

Erythromycin

The suggestion that erythromycin estolate should not be used in pregnancy (McCormack *et al.* 1977) relates to the *mother* and not to the fetus. In the treatment of genital mycoplasma infection in women over 22 weeks pregnant, erythromycin estolate caused a rise in SGOT of between 40 and 130 units in 16 of 161 subjects (10%), compared to a comparable rise in four of 168 treated with clindamycin and in three of 165 treated with placebo. There was no rise in serum bilirubin and no clinical illness, and the SGOT levels subsequently returned to normal.

Care is needed in the interpretation of these findings. It has long been believed that the estolate is more likely to cause jaundice than the stearate, but the Southampton Drug Surveillance Research Unit (1983) was unable to confirm this view, and suggested that the incidence of related jaundice is less than 1 in 1 000 and probably considerably less, and that the incidence of jaundice caused by the estolate is probably no higher than that caused by the stearate. It is of interest that there was no rise in serum bilirubin in the patients assessed by McCormack *et al.* (1977); perhaps the hepatotoxic gremlin attached to erythromycin estolate is a transient subclinical biochemical change which only very rarely causes jaundice or clinical illness. If so, it is just as likely to occur in men and non-pregnant women as in those pregnant (and seemingly as likely with the stearate as with the estolate).

There seems insufficient evidence to recommend the avoidance of erythromycin in pregnancy if this antibiotic is particularly indicated. The estolate is sometimes preferred because it is better absorbed and achieves a higher serum level than the stearate.

Sulphonamides and Trimethoprim

Folic Acid Deficiency

Because both sulphonamides and trimethoprim restrict folate availability, it has been customary to advocate avoidance during pregnancy, and Nelson and Forfar (1971) found that a higher proportion of mothers of infants with major abnormality took sulphonamides over the whole of pregnancy than mothers in a control group. However, co-trimoxazole has been widely used in pregnancy without association with fetal abnormality (Hawkins 1985), and it is not therefore strictly contra-indicated, but as a precaution, if either co-trimoxazole or tri-methroprim are given during pregnancy, folic acid should be prescribed as well in a dose of 5 mg daily.

Kernicterus

Sulphonamides given to a *neonate* displace unconjugated bilirubin from serum albumen and may cause kernicterus at bilirubin levels which would not otherwise be dangerous. Accordingly sulphonamides are not given to infants during the first six weeks of life and are similarly not given to breastfeeding mothers. It has long been advocated that sulphonamides should also be avoided in late pregnancy for the same reason, but the widespread use of co-trimoxazole in pregnancy has not been associated with neonatal kernicterus (Hawkins 1985) and this author attributes the belief to theoretical speculation.

Glucose-6-phosphate Dehydrogenase Deficiency

Sulphonamides are also avoided near term because they may cause haemolytic anaemia in the presence of this enzyme deficiency. In the United Kingdom, this rare inherited disorder is seen most often among the ethnic minorities.

Nitrofurantoin and Nalidixic Acid

Both are apparently safe in pregnancy, but are similarly avoided near term owing to the rare possibility of glucose-6-phosphate dehydrogenase deficiency.

Tetracycline

The use of tetracycline during the second half of pregnancy causes brown pigmentation of fetal decidual teeth, and in a small proportion, enamel hypoplasia. Tetracycline is also deposited in fetal bones, but evidence for its causation of fetal abnormality is less convincing than generally believed. In both the large retrospective study (Nelson and Forfar 1971) and the large prospective study (Birmingham Research Unit of the Royal College of General Practitioners 1975) the use of tetracycline was unrelated to major fetal abnormality. A single instance of multiple fetal abnormality occurring in a woman who became pregnant while taking a tetracycline long-term for acne (Corcoran and Castles 1977) cannot be ignored, but being an individual case report might come into Hawkins' (1985) category of an unjustified conclusion.

Despite the probability that tetracycline rarely causes fetal abnormality, there is adequate justification to avoid its use throughout pregnancy, and this recommendation applies also to doxycycline.

LACTATION

The Healthy Mother

All the commonly used antibiotics enter the breast milk, but problems occurring in the infant are not great. Drugs peak in the breast milk 1–4 hours after a feed (Grant and Golightly 1983), hence the dose in the milk will be lower if the mother receives her medication just before a feed.

The penicillins carry a small risk of allergy. An example (Savage 1978) is the use of intramuscular penicillin for both mother and child soon after delivery, and then the ingestion by the infant of a 'second dose' in the breast milk resulting in an allergic reaction. Cephalosporins taken by the mother may also cause an allergic reaction in the infant if the *infant* has previously received *penicillin*. The broader spectrum penicillins may also rarely cause antibiotic diarrhoea or candidiasis in the infant.

The suggestion that erythromycin might alter the infant gut flora at a time when it may be important in antibody formation (Walker 1973, Savage 1978) seems unfounded (Reilly 1983), and does not constitute a contraindication to its use.

Theoretically, tetracycline should not be given to a nursing mother, but paradoxically, staining of the secondary dentition is unlikely to occur because tetracycline binds to calcium in the breast milk, preventing absorption in the infant's intestine.

Metronidazole enters the breast milk in amounts which approach infant therapeutic levels at a maternal dose of 400 mg three times daily (Heisterberg and Branebjerg 1983). These authors are uncertain whether the infant might suffer long-term side effects at such doses, and recommend a temporary cessation of breast feeding. This is practicable with the help of a breast pump, but might be the cause of permanent cessation in some patients. A lower dose of 200 mg three times daily produces lower levels in the infant, and a short course at this dosage would probably obviate interference with breast feeding.

Sulphonamides (and co-trimoxazole) are not given to the mother during the first six weeks of the infant's life owing to the risk of kernicterus, and sulphonamides, nitrofurantoin and nalidixic acid are not given if the infant has glucose-6-phosphate dehydrogenase deficiency.

Hepatic and Renal Failure

In maternal hepatic or renal failure, the breast becomes a more important route of drug excretion, and drug levels transferred to the infant will be correspondingly higher.

NEONATES

Serious neonatal infections are treated in hospital, and owing to the immature physiology of the neonate, drugs are given parenterally during the first week of life.

Skin sepsis is perhaps the only disorder likely to require prescription by the general practitioner in the neonatal period (first four weeks), but even here caution should be exercised because the neonate may require a 'septic screen' in hospital.

After the first week, drugs may be given orally but owing to reduced urinary excretion rates should be given only twice daily. Flucloxacillin or a cephalosporin will usually be used, and dosages are based on weight.

Tetracycline is avoided in order to prevent staining of the secondary dentition, and sulphonamides, nitrofurantoin and nalidixic acid are not used in the presence of glucose-6-phosphate dehydrogenase deficiency.

The aminoglycosides will rarely if ever be prescribed in the general practice setting, but antibiotic sprays containing neomycin, e.g. Tribiotic, can be harmful. In pre-term infants the neomycin is absorbed through the skin and is ototoxic.

CHILDREN

Tetracyclines are avoided throughout childhood until the age of eight years in order to prevent brown staining of the secondary dentition. A study of extracted teeth (Kinirons 1983) indicated that tetracyclines are now used less often; the proportion of children with tetracycline deposits fell from 70% in 1973 to 14.7% in 1982.

As discussed in the relevant chapters, there are now only two indications which justify a tetracycline course in children, and neither indication is very common: the use of tetracycline for atypical pneumonia if erythromycin cannot be used or is ineffective, and the use of doxycycline for acute sinusitis.

THE ELDERLY

The elderly may exhibit impaired absorption, impared distribution and impaired elimination of a drug; the latter being caused by age-related changes in the kidney and liver. Adverse reactions are also more common and reflect a compound of altered sensitivity (a greater response than expected for a given plasma concentration), concomitant disease, polypharmacy and confusion in compliance (Royal College of Physicians 1984). A majority of adverse reactions are caused by drugs acting on the cardiovascular and central nervous systems.

With a few exceptions, antibiotics are generally free from specific problems related to age. Both tetracycline and nitrofurantoin can exacerbate renal failure, and if a tetracycline is indicated, doxycycline should be used instead. The aminoglycosides may also cause toxicity due to the impaired renal function of age, but this class of antibiotic is rarely if ever indicated in the general practice setting. The rare risk of death due to blood dyscrasias induced by co-trimoxazole is higher in the elderly than in other age groups.

Drug Interactions

Digoxin

The elderly are particularly liable to digoxin toxicity and it is therefore relevant that the additional use of an antibiotic may cause digoxin toxicity in a small proportion of patients (Lindenbaum *et al.* 1981).

Diuretics

Cephaloridine in conjunction with diuretics may enhance renal damage.

Swallowing

Bliss (1984) has emphasized that the elderly commonly have

oesophageal smooth muscle dysfunction and that antibiotics may therefore be inadequately swallowed, allowing lodgement in the oesophagus with the attendant risk of oesophageal ulcer. Elderly patients should be advised to sit up and to use an adequate amount of fluid when swallowing tablets or capsules. An alternative is to prescribe in liquid form.

In fact, the occurrence of oesophageal problems is by no means confined to the elderly. A literature review (Kikendall *et al.* 1983) revealed 26 types of drug responsible for 221 cases of oesophageal injury, and that in 54% (with a mean age of 29 years) 10 different antibiotics were responsible.

HEPATIC AND RENAL IMPAIRMENT

An individual general practitioner will rarely look after a patient with significant hepatic or renal dysfunction (apart from the 'normal' elderly), and intercurrent infection in such patients will often be treated in hospital. The safety and dosage of drugs in this circumstance, including the use of antibiotics, are detailed in the British National Formulary.

Reference has already been made to the use of doxycycline instead of tetracycline, to the avoidance of nitrofurantoin and the aminoglycosides, and to the interaction between cephaloridine and diuretics in the context of impaired renal function. Reference has also been made to the belief that erythromycin estolate causes jaundice (p. 10), and to the increased drug excretion in breast milk in maternal hepatic or renal dysfunction.

The combination of tetracycline and chlorpropamide may be hepatotoxic.

DRUG INTERACTIONS

Interaction between antibiotic and the contraceptive pill, digoxin and diuretics has already been discussed.

Asthma

The use of erythromycin in a patient already taking theophylline can result in theophylline toxicity (Prince *et al.* 1981). The clinical significance of this finding is discussed in Chapter 9.

Epilepsy

Barbiturates, phenytoin and carbamazepine enhance the metabolism of doxycycline causing reduced blood levels (Neuvonen *et al.* 1975), and in order to achieve effective blood levels a double dose is needed.

Diabetes

Sulphonamides can enhance the hypoglycaemic effect of chlorpropamide, tolbutamol and glibenclamide. The same effect is caused by chloramphenicol but this antibiotic is rarely if ever indicated in the general practice setting.

The combination of tetracycline and chlorpropamide may be hepatotoxic.

Myasthenia Gravis

The aminoglycoside antibiotics will rarely if ever be prescribed in general practice, but all impair neuromuscular conduction by inhibiting the release of acetylcholine.

Alcoholism

The use of metronidazole will cause an 'Antabuse-like' reaction due to inhibition of aldehyde dehydrogenase. Non-alcoholics are advised not to drink alcohol while taking metronidazole.

Methotrexate

Sulphonamides increase the toxicity of methotrexate by displacing it from its carrier plasma protein.

Haemostasis

The anticoagulant effect of warfarin may be potentiated by sulphonamides and nalidixic acid, owing to competition at binding sites; by any broad-spectrum antibiotic which decreases intestinal flora, and by metronidazole and chloramphenicol which inhibit the hepatic metabolism of warfarin. In these circumstances, a reduced dose of warfarin should be anticipated.

ABSORPTION

The absorption of tetracycline, and to a lesser extent minocycline, is considerably reduced by milk, iron, antacids, and zinc. The advice to swallow tetracycline capsules with water, and to stop iron or iron tonics, and to avoid antacids, is given to acne sufferers receiving long-term tetracycline, but the advice is just as relevant for the short course.

In disease, ampicillin absorption is reduced in obstructive jaundice, and co-trimoxazole is poorly absorbed in both coeliac disease and small bowel diverticulosis.

REFERENCES

Bacon, J. F. and Shenfield, G. M. (1980). Pregnancy attributable to interaction between tetracycline and oral contraceptives. *Br. Med. J.*, **280**, 293

Birmingham Research Unit of the Royal College of General Practitioners (1975). Morbidity and drugs in pregnancy. *R. Coll. Gen. Pract.*, **25**, 631–645

Bliss, M. R. (1984). Tablets and capsules that stick in the oesophagus. *J. R. Coll. Gen. Pract.*, **34**, 301

British Medical Journal (1975). Antibiotic diarrhoea. *Br. Med. J.*, **4**, 243–244

Corcoran, R. and Castles, J. M. (1977). Tetracycline for acne vulgaris and possible teratogenesis. *Br. Med. J.*, **2**, 807–808

Cunliffe, W. J. (1984). Oral contraceptives and the treatment of acne. *Novum*, **28**, August, 2–3

Dash, C. H. (1975). Penicillin allergy and the cephalosporins. *J. Antimicrobial Chemother.*, **1** (Suppl.), 107–118

Dossetor, J. (1975). Drug interactions with oral contraceptives. *Br. Med. J.*, **4**, 467–468

Fraser, I. S. and Jansen, R. P. S. (1983). Why do inadvertent pregnancies occur in oral contraceptive users? *Contraception*, **27**, 531–551

Grant, E. and Golightly, P. W. (1983). Which drugs pass into breast milk, and in what quantities? *Mims Magazine*, April 15th, 38–49

Grob, P. R. (1977). The use of erythromycin in a general practice. *Scott. Med. J.*, **22**, 405–407

Hawkins, D. F. (1985). Teratogenesis and other adverse effects on the fetus of antimicrobial drugs used in pregnancy. (In press)

Heisterberg, L. and Branebjerg, P. E. (1983). Blood and milk concentrations of metronidazole in mothers and infants. *J. Perinat. Med.*, **11**, 114–118

Kikendall, J. W., Friedman, A. C., Oyewole, M. A., Fleischer, D. and Johnson, L. F. (1983). Pill-induced oesophageal injury. *Digestive Dis. Sci.*, **28**, 174–182

Kinirons, M. J. (1983). Reduction in evidence in children's teeth of use of tetracycline. *Br. Med. J.*, **287**, 1515

Lindenbaum, J., Rund, D. G., Butter Jr., V. P., Tse-Eng, D. and Ranjan Saha, J. (1981). Inactivation of digoxin by the gut flora: reversal by antibiotic therapy. *N. Engl. J. Med.*, **305**, 789–794

McCormack, W. M., George, H., Donner, A., Kodgis, L. F., Alpert, S., Lowe, E. W. and Kass, E. H. (1977). Hepatotoxicity of erythromycin estolate during pregnancy. *Antimicrob. Agents Chemother.*, **12**, 630–635 630–635

Madden, T. A. (1977). Adverse penicillin reactions in the records of a general practice 1973 to 1975. *J. R. Coll. Gen. Pract.*, **27**, 73–77

Morgan, I. (1978). Metronidazole treatment in pregnancy. *Int. J. Gynaecol. Obstet.*, **15**, 501–502

Nelson, M. M. and Forfar, J. O. (1971). Associations between drugs administered during pregnancy and congenital abnormalities of the fetus. *Br. Med. J.*, **1**, 523–527

Neuvonen, P. J., Pentilla, O., Lehtovaara, R. and Aho, K. (1975). Effect of antiepileptic drugs on the elimination of various tetracycline derivatives. *Eur. J. Clin. Pharmacol.*, **9**, 147–154

Oswald, N. T. A. (1983). Penicillin allergy: a suspect label. *Br. Med. J.*, **287**, 265–266

Patterson, R. and Anderson, J. (1982). Allergic reactions to drugs and biologic agents. *J. Am. Med. Assoc.*, **248**, 2637–2645

Petz, L. D. (1978). Immunologic cross-reactivity between penicillins and cephalosporins: a review. *J. Infect. Dis.*, **137** (Suppl.), 74–79

Philipson, A. (1983). The use of antibiotics in pregnancy. *J. Antimicrob. Chemother.*, **12**, 101–104

Prince, R. A., Wing, D. S., Weinberger, M. M., Hendeles, L. S. and Reigelman, S. (1981). The effect of erythromycin on theophylline kinetics. *J. Allergy Clinic. Immunol.*, **68**, 427–431

Reilly, S. (1983). Personal communication.

Reimers, D., Nocke-Finck, L. and Breuer, H. (1974). Rifampicin, 'pill' do not go well together. *J. Am. Med. Assoc.*, **277**, 8

Royal College of Physicians (1984). Medication for the elderly. *J. R. Coll. Physicians, London*, **18**, January 1984

Savage, R. L. (1978). Let's not poison the breast milk! *Nursing Mirror*, **146**, 24–26

Schwartz, H. J. and Sher, T. H. (1984). Anaphylaxis to penicillin in a frozen dinner. *Ann. Allergy*, **52**, 342–343

Simmonds, J., Hodges, S., Nicol, F. and Barnett, D. (1978). Anaphylaxis after oral penicillin. *Br. Med. J.*, **2**, 1404

Southampton Drug Surveillance Research Unit (1983). Jaundice and erythromycin. *P.E.M. News*, August, No. 1, 8-9

Stockley, I. H. (1982). Antibiotics and oral contraceptive failure: an update. *Pharm. J.*, **229**, 525-528

Sullivan, T. J. (1984). *Staphylococcus aureus. N. Engl. J. Med.*, **311**, 795-796

Sullivan, T. J., Yecies, L. D., Shatz, G. S., Parker, C. W. and Wedner, H. J. (1982). Desensitization of patients allergic to penicillin using orally administered B-lactam antibiotics. *J. Allergy Clin. Immunol.*, **69**, 275-282

Teasley, D. G., Gerding, D. N., Olson, M. M., Peterson, L. R., Gebhard, R. L., Schwartz, M. J. and Lee Jr., J. T. (1983). Prospective randomised trial of metronidazole versus vancomycin for *Clostridium difficile*-associated diarrhoea and colitis. *Lancet*, 2, 1043-1046

Walker, W. A. (1973). Immunology of the gastrointestinal tract: Part 1. *J. Pediatr.*, **83**, 517-530

2
Management Principles

Respiratory illness is the commonest disorder seen in general practice, and represents the largest prospective area of antibiotic prescribing. Many of these illnesses are complex, comprising respiratory and non-respiratory features, and their full understanding involves also a knowledge of infections arising in the gastro-intestinal and urinary tracts. Many diagnoses are merely a collection of symptoms, and even if a 'diagnosis' is found, e.g. tonsillitis or otitis media, it is problematical whether this is the whole diagnosis owing to the presence of other associated illness features. The decision to prescribe can be difficult when the diagnosis is imprecise.

Diagnostic Labels

The multiplicity of symptoms and the diagnostic difficulty has led to the development of labels, but problems arise if an attempt is made to base treatment upon a diagnostic label. Upper respiratory tract infection, upper respiratory illness and corzya have little meaning, and it is unhelpful in treatment terms, to arbitrarily divide respiratory infections into upper, middle and lower respiratory illness, because cough with its attendant possibility of a chest infection is a common accompaniment of a cold, and examination of the chest is an integral part of assessing 'upper' respiratory illness.

It is easy to see how a patient with a sore and red throat, headache, runny nose and pyrexia could be labelled as having 'flu or coryza or pharyngitis (Coffman 1975), and how the doctor who uses an antibiotic for pharyngitis might treat the patient, whereas the doctor withholding an antibiotic in 'flu or coryza might not. This example clearly shows how unsatisfactory diagnostic labels can lead to differences in prescribing habits (Howie 1972).

Labels cannot be abandoned, but their use should be confined for two purposes: to communicate the broad area of disorder, and to reassure patients. A patient, for example, is greatly reassured to know that he has ' 'flu'.

Selective Antibiotic Use

The real diagnosis is a viral or bacterial infection or both, and thinking in this way enables a more intelligent treatment decision by attempting to recognize which component parts of the illness are of viral origin and which bacterial. The use of an antibiotic may then be considered if the illness contains a bacterial component. This means that in terms of antibiotic prescribing, each component part of an illness is assessed on its own merits. This ideal need not fail owing to the impossibility of immediately identifying either bacterium or virus.

Selective use of antibiotics based upon the viral/bacterial concept requires recognition that many illnesses are complex and that there is a wide overlap in symptomatology. In assessing the patient, therefore, the doctor should be prepared to find or to look for one or more of the following components: cold, cough, sore throat, tonsillitis, sinusitis, otitis media, laryngitis, croup, tracheitis, bronchitis, asthma, pneumonia, conjunctivitis, pyrexia, headache, myalgia, vomiting, diarrhoea, meningism and rash. It is then necessary to identify which component reflects a viral cause and which bacterial. Subsequent chapters will discuss the place of antibiotics in each individual illness-component, but as an example, an illness including pneumonia, sinusitis, otitis media or tonsillitis could lead to antibiotic prescription, whereas cough in the absence of chest signs would probably not. Similarly, non-specific symptoms, e.g. pyrexia, myalgia etc. are not in themselves an indication for antibiotic prescription.

In this manner, for example, a child with pyrexia, a cold, a cough, and otitis media but no other abnormality on examination could receive an antibiotic for the ear infection, whereas a similar illness comprising pyrexia, cold and cough without otitis media would not.

In practical terms, conducting a selective antibiotic policy in this way entails seeing the patient, taking a history and making an examination. This does not take long and it may seem a curious point to emphasize, yet in general practice there is an option to do less. Secondly, an adequate system of follow-up must be available. An illness is a dynamic process, and while, for example, an antibiotic may not be necessary now, the illness could change and require prescription subsequently. In a few patients, planned follow-up is justified, but in many it is neither necessary nor desirable, and the situation is best covered by ensuring the patient's awareness of the doctor's availability and willingness to see again if necessary. Finally, in assessing the patient, it is necessary to interpret his own interpretation of the illness. The word 'cold' may be used by the patient to cover anything from a slight cold to a full 'flu-like illness.

Justification for Using Antibiotics Selectively

In the broader scenario we are faced with a world-wide health problem due to the indiscriminate use of antibiotics, which are losing their efficiency owing to the spread of resistant organisms (*The Lancet* 1982).

A major hospital survey of antibiotic prescribing (Moss *et al.* 1981) showed that poor clinical decision-making in all kinds of infections led to a lot of over-prescribing, and the authors concluded that the one factor most likely to achieve improvement was the critical faculty of the clinician. The general practitioner has the freedom to develop this faculty, and much of the responsibility is his own. The most useful practical help is to understand more fully the nature of the illnesses he is treating.

Beyond the broader issues, the indiscriminate use of antibiotics in general practice can cause more immediate problems. A prescription given routinely may take the place of advice which is necessary whether an antibiotic is given or not. A late night call, for example, can come from a parent whose child had been given an antibiotic that same day, but was inadequately advised about what might happen that night. More ominously, perhaps, routine prescription might engender the view that there is little point in examining the patient at all, encouraging telephone diagnosis, resulting in a poor standard of care and eliminating once and for all any chance of learning the nature and pattern of each illness. The advice most needed by the patient is a forecast of what may happen and how then to cope, and in order to impart this information, knowledge of illness patterns is necessary.

A further problem concerns antibiotic side effects. To add diarrhoea to a child already ill is at best an unwelcome occurrence, but is particularly unkind if the antibiotic was not necessary in the first place. Additionally, some patients will develop penicillin allergy and to acquire this state unnecessarily is more than unfortunate.

In opposition to selective antibiotic use is the belief that withholding antibiotics creates more work, and while this particular point has not been proven, Howie and Hutchison (1978) have shown in a retrospective study that large scale antibiotic prescribing did not *save* work, and suggested therefore a move away from prescribing and towards educating.

It is not difficult to see why high antibiotic prescribing fails to save work. If a patient or child's mother believes that every cold or similar illness requires an antibiotic, they will return every time such an illness occurs in order to obtain the 'necessary' prescription (Howie 1975). If, however, after experiencing one or two consultations which result in explanation and advice, but no prescription, it is probable that subsequent minor illnesses will be self-treated, and advice sought only if self-treatment fails or if the illness is more severe. There are no figures to support the view that reduced antibiotic prescribing results in a lower initial consultation rate, but experience suggests that this is so, and Marsh (1977) found that selective prescribing gave time to practise a better quality of medicine. The belief that selective antibiotic use increases work is therefore unfounded.

The sort of problem which can be caused by overprescribing is exemplified by the late evening visit request from a distraught mother, whose child had been seen earlier that day. The child had a cold, a cough and vomiting, and had been given three bottles of medicine: an antibiotic, a cough medicine and phenergan (for the vomiting). The mother was distraught because the child was unable to keep any of the medicines down owing to the vomiting, and she reasonably thought they were essential because they had been prescribed. None of the drugs were in fact necessary, and what the mother needed was advice on the nature of the illness, advice on the self-limiting character of the vomiting and advice on how to cope.

Variations in Antibiotic Prescribing

While selective antibiotic use based upon a viral/bacterial understanding of the illness represents a reasonable approach, this general policy may become waived in two opposing directions. In one direction, antibiotics may be given in the absence of a bacterial component. A reason for this is prescription in good faith but on a questionable indication, and examples are the child with a 'bad' or 'chesty' cough in the absence of apparent chest infection, or if there is uncertainty of the extent to which a bacterial element may contribute, e.g. laryngitis or croup.

A further reason for questionable prescribing is the existence of a psycho-social situation in relation to the illness. This concerns the orientation of the general practitioner more to the patient, as compared with orientation more to the illness in hospital medicine (Howie 1978). Howie (1976) has suggested how the awareness of a social circumstance in addition to a clinical illness can influence prescribing and result in a higher incidence of antibiotic use. Another form of psycho-social prescribing concerns treating a child unnecessarily in order to placate a stressed mother (Howie and Bigg 1980). This situation can be managed without unnecessary prescription, but it involves a willingness to reassure in practical terms by seeing the child daily or even more often, and also a willingness to visit should the need arise. If the child is initially examined, genuine concern shown, advice given and a positive follow-up arrangement made, then even the more anxious mother will acknowledge the direct comment that it is not really right to give the child an unnecessary antibiotic just to keep her happy.

Such an approach does take time, but the learning and confidence gained by the mother in seeing the illness follow the advised pattern and her child getting better without an antibiotic will alter her subsequent behaviour, and lead to a lower consultation rate. Further, the time spent has a longer-term benefit as well, because it is likely (Howie 1983) that patterns of expectation and behaviour created in one generation will pass to the next.

Rarely, it may be necessary to prescribe unnecessarily and accept defeat. Such patients include those with limited intelligence, the emotionally disturbed menopausal woman and the patient who 'knows his rights'.

In the opposite direction, an antibiotic may be withheld despite the presence of a bacterial component and this aspect of antibiotic prescribing creates the most argument. It has to be acknowledged that many bacterial infections can recover without antibiotic use, but how far should the doctor go in withholding prescription? Even pneumonia can recover spontaneously.

The answers may lie in a better understanding of the individual disorders, but the point should be made that if a substantial reduction in unnecessary antibiotic use is going to be achieved, the bulk of this reduction is going to occur in the much larger field of uncomplicated colds, coughs and 'flu-like illnesses which do have a viral cause. It could be less relevant to make too big an issue about withholding antibiotics in smaller groups of patients with an acute illness and a likely bacterial cause, e.g. tonsillitis and otitis media.

Training the Patient

The fundamental rule is that no prescription shall be issued unless the patient is seen. If an antibiotic is considered unnecessary when a patient is seen, an explanation is given on the relative role of virus and bacterium, and advice given on the expected pattern of the illness; on the management of pyrexia if relevant, and on simple home remedies, e.g. antipyretics, steam, and what to eat and drink. Some of this advice, of course, will also be given if an antibiotic *is* prescribed. The doctor should not be afraid to say that there is no specific treatment, and that the disease has to run its course, and the general message to impart is that the doctor will always be willing to check a patient, but will prescribe only if necessary. As always, the availability of a follow-up check should be seen to be offered willingly.

The initiation of such a programme in a practice which has previously had looser prescribing routines may cause initial consternation, and may involve home visiting which would not otherwise have been undertaken, and it takes time to give a convincing explanation. The initial work load is undoubtedly increased, but as previously discussed, is self-limiting and pays dividends.

The excellent and comprehensive training programme instituted by Marsh (1977) demonstrates all these points. The patient tended to declare the real problem, e.g. psychiatric or marital; many patients had anxieties about drugs and were pleased that prescription was not necessary; a mother would bring her child to be checked without expectation of prescription, and a better standard of practice occurred because absence of automatic prescription led to a more careful examination.

Another approach is to issue the patient with a booklet on how to cope and when to call the doctor (Morrell *et al.* 1980, Roberts *et al.* 1983), but many general practitioners would prefer to train patients personally, and some would feel that detriment could arise from delay in seeking advice.

The Doctor's Job

Now at last, the proper role of the doctor is beginning to emerge. The general practitioner is many things. He is guide, philosopher and friend; he has a continuing responsibility for the patient in both the prevention and treatment of disease, and has the opportunity to see the patient as a whole person in the context of his family and social structure, but in the field of respiratory illness and in pure clinical terms, his job is to see, to examine, to assess and to advise. Beyond this he will sometimes also prescribe, but his prescription should usually be confined to drugs with a specific purpose.

Training the Doctor

Much that has been said relating to patient training applies also to the doctor because he has to implement such training.

Advice to the patient is necessary whether an antibiotic is given or not, and an awareness of this need is most acute when a doctor is on duty for the night. During the daytime before such a night, the doctor may be most particular in giving advice on what to expect and how to cope, in order to avoid being called out during the night. That the stimulus for such advice may have an ulterior motive does not matter; the important point is that the doctor learns the *need* for giving advice.

In particular, it is the doctor's responsibility to train himself in an understanding of the nature and pattern of each illness. Examples are numerous. It is useful to know that the onset of a cough in a 'flu-like illness is sometimes delayed; that the acute phase of ' 'flu' may occur at the start or in the middle of the whole illness; that the pyrexia in measles usually persists for 24 hours beyond the time of onset of the rash. To know the expected duration of pyrexia in different illnesses is fundamental, and it is useful to know for how long crepitations will be heard in pneumonia, and what might emerge (and when) from a child with unexplained pyrexia, and for how long the child with a cough will continue to cough, and so on.

Knowledge of this sort is of immense value to the doctor. *Firstly*, it gives him confidence in managing an illness, and this confidence is always recognized by the patient and is reassuring. *Secondly*, it enables the doctor to give realistic advice and in particular to give an outline of what might happen and how then to cope. These two points are well exemplified by children with unexplained pyrexia, when occasionally it may be three or four days before a diagnosis is reached. Retention of parental confidence when the child is ill and no specific treatment is yet being given requires both knowledge and confidence by the doctor. Its lack can result in management failure; the mother takes fright and rushes the child unnecessarily to hospital. *Thirdly*, the doctor will be able to recognize a variation from the expected pattern which may indicate a complication. An example is recrudescence of pyrexia or persistence of pyrexia beyond the expected time, which in a 'flu-like illness might indicate a complicating pneumonia. *Finally*, knowledge of common illness patterns will enable the doctor to recognize more readily the occasional unusual illness.

While books and medical journals may offer a guide, much of this learning has to be self-taught. A follow-up visit can be as beneficial to the doctor as to the patient, and learning is aided by what is written in the patient's records. A terse comment like 'coryza', 'upper respiratory illness', ''flu' or 'bronchitis' is useless as a learning method and is also useless in day to day management because both detail and duration of the illness could merge into vagueness. It is far better to record specific symptoms and clinical findings in chronological order, both initially and on follow-up. In this manner, the nature and pattern of different illnesses will be learned, and in day to day management a better understanding of the illness can be achieved.

REFERENCES

Coffman, D. A. (1975). The case for the use of antibiotics in upper respiratory infections. *Update*, **10**, 1345-1348

Howie, J. G. R. (1972). Diagnosis - the Achilles heel? *J. R. Coll. Gen. Pract.*, **22**, 310-315

Howie, J. G. R. (1975). The case against use of antibiotics in upper respiratory tract illness. *Update*, **10**, 1351-1353

Howie, J. G. R. (1976). Clinical judgement and antibiotic use in general practice. *Br. Med. J.*, **2**, 1061-1064

Howie, J. G. R. (1978). The art and the epidemiologist. *J. R. Coll. Gen. Pract.*, **28**, 71-77

Howie, J. G. R. (1983). Antibiotic use in general practice. *Update*, **27**, 193-196

Howie, J. G. R. and Bigg, A. R. (1980). Family trends in psychotropic and antibiotic prescribing in general practice. *Br. Med. J.*, **280**, 836-838

Howie, J. G. R. and Hutchison, K. R. (1978). Antibiotics and respiratory illness in general practice: prescribing policy and work load. *Br. Med. J.*, **2**, 1342

Lancet, The (1982). Worldwide antibiotic misuse. Conference report. **2**, 29

Marsh, G. N. (1977). Curing minor illness in general practice. *Br. Med. J.*, **2**, 1267–1269

Morrell, D. C., Avery, A. J. and Watkins, C. J. (1980). Management of minor illness. *Br. Med. J.*, **280**, 769–771

Moss, F., McNicol, M. W., McSwiggan, D. A. *et al.* (1981). Survey of antibiotic prescribing in a district general hospital. *Lancet*, **2**, 349–352, 407–409, 461–462

Roberts, C. R., Imrey, P. B., Turner, J. D., Hosokawa, M. C. and Alster, J. M. (1983). Reducing physician visits for colds through consumer education. *J. Am. Med. Assoc.*, **250**, 1986–1989

3
Pyrexia

Febrile Convulsions – Delirium – Rigors – Symptomatic Management of Pyrexia – Antibiotic Use

The classically defined patterns of pyrexia are seldom seen now, and in general practice today the pyrexial patterns which matter are those occurring in relation to the commoner illnesses, e.g. influenza, the 'flu-like illness, 'upper respiratory illness' and the exanthems.

Patients with a raised temperature will usually exhibit certain symptoms. Adults tend to feel cold, 'hug the fire', shiver, or feel 'hot and cold' and occasionally will faint. Children react in a different way. They lose their appetite, 'lie about' and sleep more. The child who presents with a story of having slept all the afternoon will invariably be pyrexial.

The diurnal temperature swing in a pyrexial patient is a common phenomenon, and it is sometimes useful to advise the patient that the temperature will tend to come down in the morning, and go up again in the afternoon, evening and night. The swing is also of relevance to the assessment of a patient who may not seem to be hot at the time actually seen, and in this circumstance, the patient's report of the symptoms of pyrexia, e.g. the previous evening or night, can help to establish whether the patient has a pyrexial illness.

FEBRILE CONVULSIONS

Febrile convulsions occur in children aged 1–5 years and mostly in those aged 1–3 years. About two in every 100 children will have a fit in the first five years of life, and about a quarter of these children will have more than one fit (Stokes et al. 1977). In children under the age of six months, a fit is likely to have a specific cause and the infant should be admitted to hospital. Such a fit should neither be labelled nor managed as a febrile convulsion (Jolly 1981).

The febrile convulsion occurs early in the febrile illness, and contrary to popular belief does not commonly occur at the height of the temperature, but usually develops earlier, and may occur so early in the illness that it is not yet apparent that the child has pyrexia.

Predisposing Factors

A child with manifest neurological disease may have a convulsion when pyrexial, but the commonly seen febrile convulsion occurs in children who are apparently normal, and the predisposition is a lowered convulsive threshold. Genetic factors play a part (Jolly 1981) and there is also evidence that an abnormal pregnancy or birth history will predispose to febrile convulsions (Wallace 1972).

The triggering factor is the fever itself, and is not a specific manifestation of infection by any particular agent. A wide range of viral infections are associated (Poole and Tobin 1973, Stokes et al. 1977), and the cause will be whichever pathogen is endemic or epidemic in the community at the time. In Nigeria, the commonest cause is malaria.

Management

A child will sometimes be taken direct to hospital, but if the general practitioner is involved he has various options. In one situation, the fit will be over by the time the doctor arrives. If this was the first fit, if it was brief and if the child is now apparently well, then it is hoped that no further fits will occur, and attention is given to managing the triggering pyrexial illness. This illness is assessed, managed and treated strictly according to its own needs. Antibiotics are used selectively and will not always be necessary.

If the child is actually fitting while the doctor is present, then if it is the first fit there is no need for interference and the doctor waits for it to cease, ensuring that the child is on his side in order to avoid the inhalation of vomit. The doctor should then remain in the household for a short while longer in case a second fit should rapidly follow, and in its absence may then leave the house, but should return an hour or so later to assess and manage the pyrexial illness. Clinical examination immediately after a fit is best avoided.

Sometimes, however, the fit does not cease quickly, or this may already be an immediate second one, and in either of these situations rectal diazepam should be given, and immediate transfer to hospital arranged. Rectal diazepam is given in a dose of 0.5 mg/kg, and outside hospital the dose should not exceed 5 mg. The diazepam used may either be part of the ampoule designed for parenteral use, or the commercially available rectal diazepam solution (Stesolid), containing 2 mg or 4 mg per ml in tubes of 2.5 ml. When the child reaches hospital, further diazepam may be needed and given intravenously.

Should a child have a second fit much later (months or a year or two later), this episode is managed as a 'first' fit as already outlined, but subsequent paediatric referral is advisable.

Prevention

The use of phenobarbitone twice daily for 48 hours to 'cover' the immediate pyrexial illness is ineffective owing to its slow absorption (6–18 hours), and although sodium valproate is absorbed faster, its full therapeutic effect may take longer. In practice, the use of anti-convulsants on a short-term basis is unhelpful.

On a longer-term basis, the mother will invariably ask if there is any way of preventing a further convulsion when the child next has a temperature. Rectal diazepam would probably be effective and could be left with the mother for prophylactic use, but the real problems are that febrile convulsions tend to occur so early in the illness that the mother is often unaware that a pyrexial illness is developing, and secondly, that despite instruction, the mother will commonly be reluctant to give any drug without current medical advice when the next pyrexial illness does become evident.

The only valid method of prevention is to use an anticonvulsant drug in full dosage on a long-term basis, and a decision for use should be made by a paediatrician because assessment includes EEG. Factors tending to justify such drug use are a prolonged fit, a family history of febrile convulsions, more than one convulsion, and the possibility of epilepsy. In the absence of believed epilepsy, the drug is usually stopped again after two years free of fits, and by the age of five years the tendency to febrile convulsions will cease.

Long-term phenobarbitone causes irritability and hyperactivity, and either sodium valproate or less commonly carbamazepine are more suitable drugs. During long-term treatment the child is seen and weighed every three months in order to consider dose alterations in relation to growth.

DELIRIUM

Delirium in association with pyrexia is seen in the older child, occurring most commonly in those aged between five and 10 years, but may be seen in a child as young as three years. Delirium occurs at the height of a high temperature, and in this way differs from the very early occurrence of the febrile convulsion, but delirium does, however, also occur early in the illness and nearly always becomes manifest during the first night of the pyrexia. It is less common for delirium to occur on a second or subsequent night, but delirium has been seen in an eight year old child with measles on the fourth day of pyrexia when the rash was emerging. Delirium at this late stage is understandable because the pyrexia in a child with measles is highest just before the rash appears.

The incidence of delirium (about two in every 100 pyrexial children) is similar to the incidence of the febrile convulsion, but it is not clear why any particular child should become delirious. The infective cause of the high temperature is most commonly tonsillitis or a 'flu-like illness, but delirium can occur with a high temperature from any cause.

Management entails tepid-sponging and/or the use of a fan which results in a small temperature reduction and restores normality. Should a child of this age-group be seen during the daytime when early in a pyrexial illness, the parents can be warned of the possibility of delirium during the night, and advised how to cope. The cause of the infection is treated strictly according to its needs. Antibiotics are used selectively and are not always necessary.

RIGORS

The rigor is suffered by adults, but is similar to the febrile convulsions and delirium occurring early in a pyrexial illness. The immediate cause is a rapid rise in temperature, which causes skin vessels to constrict in an attempt to conserve heat, and then, because the body surface feels cold, violent shivering ensues. Colloquially known as 'the ague', the patient with a rigor shakes all over, and if on a bed, the bed shakes as well.

Any infection causing a rapid temperature rise may cause a rigor, and the pathological cause is a transient bacteraemia, viraemia or parasitaemia. The classical and best known cause is malaria, but the two commonest causes presenting to the general practitioner are a urinary tract infection or an influenzal illness (influenza itself or a 'flu-like illness). Less common causes include pneumonia, cholangitis, and now, with an ageing population, acute bacterial endocarditis (Welsby 1977).

The prime aim in management is to expeditiously diagnose the cause and to initiate treatment according to its needs. The rigor is self-limiting, but the patient is made more comfortable if temporarily kept warm.

SYMPTOMATIC MANAGEMENT OF PYREXIA

Is it necessary to 'bring the temperature down' and what advice should the doctor give?

The Mechanism of Fever

Endogenous pyrogens liberated by mononuclear phagocytic cells (Wood 1984) in response to a bacterial or viral stimulus act on the hypothalamus causing a raised thermoregulatory set-point. Kluger (1980) suggests that an endogenous cryogen may also exist and that fluctuations in temperature could involve an interplay between pyrogen and cryogen.

The Benefits of Fever

Fever in disease is beneficial. Human host defences are enhanced, and in animal experiments an elevation of body temperature enhances survival rate in induced infection. In evolutionary terms, fever in disease would not have been selectively retained for so long and in so many species if it had no advantage (Kluger 1980).

The Dangers of Fever

Hyperpyrexia denoted by a temperature of over 41 °C is dangerous, but rarely are such high temperatures caused by the bacterial or viral infections commonly seen in medical practice. Possibly the only exceptions are babies who are allowed to become overheated by excessive clothing or by a particularly warm environment, and can then die from febrile apnoea, representing the younger infant's fatal equivalent of a febrile convulsion (Stanton 1984). The clinical presentation is that of a cot death, and there is commonly evidence of both physical overheating and a bacterial or viral infection.

Temperature Reduction

It is commonly argued that the temperature should be brought down in small children in order to prevent febrile convulsions, but the validity of this argument is questionable because febrile convulsions commonly occur very early in the illness, before the temperature has had a chance to rise much. It makes greater sense to advocate temperature reduction in children aged 5-10 years in order to prevent delirium, which *does* occur at the height of a high temperature, and also to prevent overheating in babies with viral infections in order to avoid fatal febrile apnoea.

It has to be concluded that while temperature reduction, or the avoidance of overheating, is sometimes indicated as stated, temperature reduction tends not to be necessary in a majority of patients.

This conclusion needs to be evaluated in the light of decades of tradition. Nearly every household has aspirin, aspirin compounds, or paracetamol in the medicine cupboard, and the mothers of children widely believe that temperature should be reduced. It is also the experience of both general practitioners and parents that the well-being of a pyrexial child can be improved by aspirin. Further, in clinical situations where arguments are presented to withhold antibiotics, and training is given to enhance self-help, it is paradoxical to then recommend avoidance of antipyretic drugs which are the mainstay of self-help.

Realistically it has to be accepted that antipyretics will continue to be used, but the important point is to ensure that no danger will ensue from their use and it is in this area that advice and patient training can be given.

Aspirin or Paracetamol (or neither)?

Aspirin, or components containing it, should be avoided in those known to have indigestion or peptic ulceration owing to the risk of gastric haemorrhage, and standard doses of aspirin are avoided in the elderly for the same reason, but the small daily dose given to prevent cerebral haemorrhage does not seem to cause trouble. A very small proportion of patients are allergic to aspirin, and may develop asthma.

In pregnancy, aspirin is better avoided during the second and third trimester. Aspirin in high doses during this period of time may cause post-maturity and prolonged labour owing to inhibition of prostaglandin synthesis, and can also cause a prolonged bleeding time owing to impaired platelet aggregation which increases the risk of ante- and post-partum haemorrhage. Haemorrhage in the infant may also occur (Perris 1983). If a simple analgesic or antipyretic is needed during pregnancy, paracetamol is preferable. The much smaller dose used to prevent placental infarction in order to reduce the incidence of pre-eclamptic toxaemia, intra-uterine growth retardation and stillbirth (Beaufils et al. 1985) did not cause abnormal bleeding in either mother or child.

During lactation, either paracetamol or an occasional dose of aspirin may be used, but larger doses of aspirin used more regularly should be avoided, again owing to the risk of impaired platelet function.

On a wider plane, Stanley et al. (1975) have demonstrated increased virus shedding in adults infected with rhinovirus and treated with aspirin, suggesting that aspirin might not be the ideal drug for home use in respiratory viral infection, and that such use might enhance the spread of infection.

A drawback to the use of aspirin in small children is the risk of inadvertent therapeutic toxicity (Craig et al. 1966). Children under the age of two years have a greater susceptibility to salicylates. Aspirin should not be used at all under the age of twelve months and is better avoided under the age of two years. Paracetamol would seem to be safe in small children, given in recommended doses, but empirically should not be given under the age of three months.

Reye's syndrome

A shadow has been cast on the use of aspirin in children and teenagers owing to its possible contribution to Reye's syndrome. This syndrome (Khan 1983, Addy 1983, Mowat 1983) comprises cerebral oedema and fatty infiltration of the liver, and presents as profuse vomiting three or four days after a viral illness, and then progresses through mental confusion with possibly convulsions or delirium, to coma. There is an associated hypoglycaemia. The prodromal illness is usually Influenza B or chicken pox or a diarrhoeal illness. Reye's syndrome is very rare, and a causative role for aspirin is by no means proven (Glasgow 1984).

To the general practitioner who has never seen the syndrome, there may seem little justification in withholding aspirin, but it could be sensible in one's day to day management and training of patients, to gradually veer away from aspirin and move towards paracetamol.

The Avoidance of Overheating

The avoidance of overheating relates primarily to babies and small children. Excessive clothes are removed, and in the absence of draughts or a frankly cold atmosphere, it is better to remove all clothing. Unnecessary bed clothes are removed at night, remembering that it can become colder at 1.00 am or 2.00 am, when replacement of a blanket may be necessary. Atmospheric heating is reduced if excessive, and an attempt made to adequately ventilate without draughts.

These measures would tend to be undertaken if the baby or small child *is* hot, and rightly so, but the findings of Stanton (1984) indicate that if a cot death due to overheating is to be prevented, the advice on avoidance of overheating will sometimes need to be given *before* the child is obviously hot, when initially seen for any particular viral or bacterial infection, e.g. during the day or in the evening.

Physical Cooling

This method of temperature reduction may be undertaken in a patient of any age. Tepid sponging is the classic method, and entails sponging most of the body surface, e.g. face, back and limbs, with a wet flannel which is cooler than the patient but not cold. The skin surface is then dried and any necessary clothing replaced. The degree of temperature reduction achieved is modest, and it may be necessary to sponge more than once because it has long been known that the temperature of a febrile patient returns again to its original elevated level after physical cooling. Sponging with ice-cold water or alcohol achieves a greater temperature reduction, but causes excessive discomfort and shivering (Steele *et al.* 1970), and should not therefore be used.

An alternative method of cooling is to use a small electric fan or an electric blow-heater without the heat turned on.

Advice to the Patient

Advice concerning the avoidance of overheating, physical cooling and the use of antipyretic drugs follows the guidelines already discussed. The doctor should usually not *prescribe* antipyretic drugs, because his prescription leads a patient to believe that it is an essential drug. An example is the pyrexial asthmatic child for whom salbutamol syrup and paracetamol elixir were prescribed. The mother gave the paracetamol first and then withheld the salbutamol because she thought it might react adversely with the paracetamol. Antipyretic drugs should be purchased, and the doctor should comment, in any particular instance, on the advisability of use. If an essential drug *is* prescribed, the doctor can advise that his drug will not 'fight' with the home remedy. The example given emphasises yet again that problems may ensue from unnecessary prescribing.

Hot children will not eat, and the mother should be reassured that this is a temporary phase and of no consequence. An anoxic atmosphere might be a contributory factor in the causation of febrile convulsions, and in the winter therefore, if a coal fire is used, a window should be left slightly open in order to allow adequate ventilation.

ANTIBIOTIC USE

Pyrexia *per se* is not an indication for antibiotic use. Antibiotics are prescribed selectively dependent upon cause and individual illness features.

REFERENCES

Addy, D.P. (1983). Cold comfort for hot children. *Br. Med. J.*, **286**, 1163–1164

Beaufils, M., Uzan, S., Donsimoni, R. and Colau, J.C. (1985). Prevention of pre-eclampsia by early antiplatelet therapy. *Lancet*, **1**, 840–842

Craig, J.O., Ferguson, I.C. and Syme, J. (1966). Infants, toddlers, and aspirin. *Br. Med. J.*, **1**, 757–761

Glasgow, J. F. T. (1984). Clinical features and prognosis of Reye's Syndrome. *Arch. Dis. Child.*, **59**, 230–235

Jolly, H. (1981). *Diseases of Children*, p. 366. (Oxford, London, Edinburgh, Boston and Melbourne: Blackwell Scientific Publications)

Khan, N. (1983). Reye's Syndrome. *Br. Med. J.*, **287**, 128

Kluger, M. J. (1980). Fever. *Pediatrics*, **66**, 720–724

Mowat, A. P. (1983). Reye's Syndrome: 20 years on. *Br. Med. J.*, **286**, 1999–2001

Perris, B. W. (1983). The right analgesic to recommend for the pregnant woman. *Mims Magazine*, **May**, 86–93

Poole, P. M. and Tobin, J. O'H. (1973). Viral and epidemiological findings in MRC/PHLS surveys of respiratory disease in hospital and general practice. *Postgrad. Med. J.*, **49**, 778–787

Stanley, E. D., Jackson, G. G., Panusarn, C., Rubenis, M. and Dirda, V. (1975). Increased virus shedding with aspirin treatment of rhinovirus infection. *J. Am. Med. Assoc.*, **231**, 1248–1251

Stanton, A. N. (1984). Overheating and cot death. *Lancet*, **2**, 1199–1201

Steele, R. W., Tanaka, P. T., Lara, R. P. and Bass, J. W. (1970). Evaluation of sponging and of oral antipyretic therapy to reduce fever. *J. Pediatr.*, **77**, 824–829

Stokes, M. J., Downham, M. A. P. S., Webb, J. K. G., McQuillin, J. and Gardner, P. S. (1977). Viruses and febrile convulsions. *Arch. Dis. Child.*, **52**, 129–133

Wallace, S. J. (1972). Aetiological aspects of febrile convulsions. *Arch. Dis. Child.*, **47**, 171–177

Welsby, P. D. (1977). Infective endocarditis – a retrospective study. *The Practitioner*, **218**, 382–387

Wood, M. J. (1984). Fever. *Med. Int.*, **2**, 9–15

4

Sore Throat, Tonsillitis and Pharyngitis

Definition – The Non-inflamed Sore Throat – The Inflamed Throat – Referral for Tonsillectomy

For years tonsillitis has been shadowed by the risk of rheumatic fever, and antibiotic treatment has been dictated by the need to eradicate the streptococcus. It is only in recent years with reduction in rheumatic fever incidence to rarity, that tonsillitis has been looked at more as a disorder in its own right. Consequent upon this, the place of antibiotic treatment has also been questioned.

Sore throat is the most controversial area in the whole field of respiratory illness. Particular reasons include the use of the symptomatic term 'sore throat' as a diagnosis; confusion in terminology between 'tonsillitis' and 'pharyngitis'; inadequate recognition of the non-inflamed sore throat, and difficulties of interpretation between viral and bacterial causes. These latter difficulties are compounded partly by the erroneous assumption that absence of a bacterial isolation automatically means a viral cause, and partly by lack of knowledge.

Discussion of the subject will be based upon the different types of sore throat as shown in Figure 4.1, the point of departure being a clinical differentiation by naked eye examination between patients who have an inflamed throat and those who do not.

DEFINITION

Sore Throat a Symptom

There is widespread failure to appreciate that many patients with a sore throat do not have either tonsillitis or pharyngitis. The term sore throat

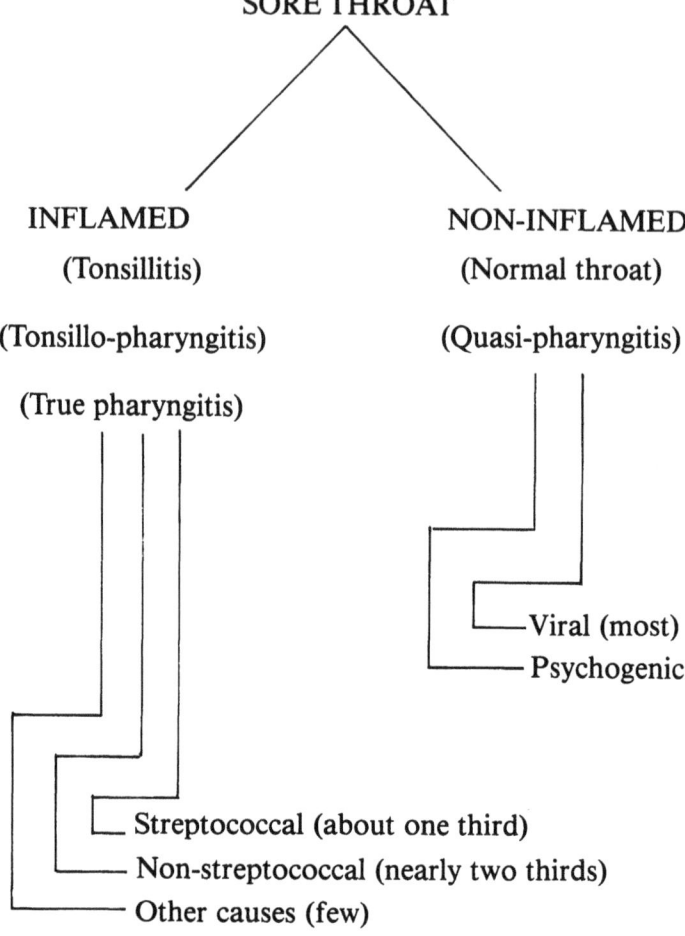

Figure 4.1 Types of sore throat

is by definition symptomatic yet is widely used as a diagnosis, and this incorrect usage creates confusion. While eminent and respected members of the medical profession continue to use the term as a diagnosis, confusion will persist.

Tonsillitis or Pharyngitis?

The two terms are often used synonymously, and this situation is unlikely to change because it is the custom in some countries to call tonsillitis pharyngitis. The only realistic way round this dilemma is to define whether the throat is inflamed or non-inflamed. What is particularly wrong is to mistake the normal redness of the throat for pharyngitis (quasi-pharyngitis), and then feel compelled to prescribe an antibiotic because the word pharyngitis means inflammation.

True pharyngitis is represented by tonsillo-pharyngitis; by the uncommon, deep red, angry, oedematous inflammation of the faucial pillars, and by the rarely seen inflammation and lymphoid hyperplasia of the posterior pharyngeal wall.

THE NON-INFLAMED SORE THROAT

Roughly half the total incidence of patients with a sore throat will have a throat which looks normal.

Cause and Incidence

The non-inflamed sore throat is seen most commonly in adults but does occur in children. By far the commonest cause is a viral infection and the illnesses are typically 'colds and coughs' and 'flu-like illnesses. Roughly half the incidence of adults with an enterovirus 'flu (Echo or Coxsackie virus) will have a sore throat, most being non-inflamed, and nearly all the respiratory virus 'flu illnesses do so. Of necessity, therefore, the incidence of soreness without visible inflammation rises during an outbreak of a viral infection, and reaches its zenith during an influenza epidemic. The mechanism of soreness is probably viral infiltration of the naso-pharynx.

A much smaller proportion of patients have a psychogenic cause for their normal-looking sore throat. The symptom has its origin in anxiety or depression, and the patient is usually a middle-aged woman who invariably presents having already had the sore throat for about two weeks.

Supporting Evidence for the Existence of the Non-inflamed Sore Throat

The non-inflamed sore throat has only recently been described as an entity (Everett 1979a), but supporting evidence for its existence comes from the findings and comments of Moffet *et al.* (1968), Feery *et al.* (1976), Bridges-Webb (1977) and Shaheen (1983). It is evident that the term pharyngitis is being used by some to denote the inflamed throat, and by others erroneously to describe what is surely the normal throat.

Further evidence comes from a Combined Scottish study (1975) which indicated a negative clinical prediction of streptococcal infection in sore throats occurring with colds and influenza. This prediction is as expected because the incidence of a 'flu illness with an inflamed sore throat is much lower than the incidence with a non-inflamed sore throat.

Significance of the Non-inflamed Sore Throat

Antibiotics are rarely necessary in treatment (see next section), but the significance of the non-inflamed sore throat goes further than this. In studies of tonsillitis, inclusion of non-inflamed sore throats will give an erroneous impression of a low streptococcal incidence, and an adverse impression of antibiotic efficacy. To see quoted as recently as 1982 that the 'streptococcal incidence in tonsillitis and acute sore throat varies between 5 and 30%' demonstrates the misunderstandings that can arise. Studies confined to the inflamed throat show a consistent streptococcal incidence of between 30 and 40%.

The non-inflamed sore throat has relevance also to the view that because many people with tonsillitis do not seek medical advice, it is perhaps pointless treating those who do. Valkenberg et al. (1971) concluded that only 8.7% of patients suffering from a streptococcal sore throat visited their physician. This figure is widely quoted, but the method of sampling on which their calculation was based involved asking the patient if there had been a sore throat in the previous month, and must surely have included some with non-inflamed sore throats. A similar comment can be made about the findings of Evans et al. (1982), who concluded that under 16% of those with streptococcal tonsillitis sought advice. Their sampling method was symptomatic only and was conducted by post.

While there will always be some people who do not readily seek medical advice, it is probable that a majority with tonsillitis (inflamed throat) do so.

Future research on throat infection should clarify exactly what is being studied.

Antibiotic Use

The non-inflamed sore throat does not require antibiotic use because there is no visible inflammation and because the cause of the soreness is viral. There are, however, two uncommon clinical situations in which antibiotics are justified.

The Bypass Phenomenon

First described by Dr G. I. Watson, the infecting organism bypasses the throat and causes significant tonsillar node enlargement. The throat looks normal, but the clinical picture in all other aspects is that expected in tonsillitis. Griffiths (1979) reports the same phenomenon under the name tonsillar adenitis.

Recurrent Tonsillitis

A majority of children with frequently recurring tonsillitis will of course have an obviously inflamed throat each time an attack occurs, but occasionally, despite sore throat and pyrexia, the tonsils, although enlarged and rugged-looking, appear non-inflamed. These occasional instances should be recognized as having a bacterial cause.

THE INFLAMED THROAT

Patients with an inflamed throat have tonsillitis, tonsillo-pharyngitis, or true pharyngitis as already defined.

Age Incidence

Two thirds are under the age of 20 years, and most of the remainder under 40. The highest incidence occurs in those aged 5-10 years (25%) and the incidence then gradually decreases through teenage and adult life. The child under five years of age may also suffer from tonsillitis, certainly down to the age of three years, and occasionally two years. Tonsillitis *does* occur in infants under the age of one year, but it is problematical whether very small children and infants are commonly affected. Clinical experience suggests not. The particular difficulty concerns diagnosis because the crying and struggling which may be associated with the use of a tongue depressor in a young child causes the throat to become congested, rendering diagnosis uncertain.

A general practitioner will need to examine a child several times for various reasons between the ages of two and five years, and a valid assessment is aided by a child's continuing co-operation. This co-operation could be vitiated by unpleasant experiences with a tongue depressor, and unless the clinical situation makes it imperative to see the throat in those under two years of age (e.g. a particularly high temperature or no obvious diagnosis), then it could be wiser not to look.

Clinical Features and Causes

Streptococcal and Non-Streptococcal Tonsillitis

There is no reliable method of differentiating streptococcal from non-streptococcal tonsillitis on clinical grounds. Studies which have attempted to define positive or negative predictions of streptococcal infection, or have devised scoring systems, are able to indicate a trend either for or against streptococcal infection, but these studies have tended to embrace the whole field of sore throat. Of necessity, therefore, non-inflamed sore throats would have been included in the assessment, and it is possibly for this reason that such trends are evident. If study is confined to inflamed throats, close scrutiny of all clinical parameters serves only to demonstrate the remarkable similarity between the two types of infection. For this reason clinical features are described under the joint heading.

Clinical Presentation

The commonest presentation, typically in a child, is a combination of sore throat and high temperature, sometimes with headache and sometimes vomiting. Symptomatically, this clinical picture could be recognized also as a non-respiratory viral illness in which the throat could be non-inflamed. The only way to determine whether tonsillitis is or is not present, is to look at the throat.

The same situation occurs in adults, when a combination of sore throat (symptom), high temperature, headache and generalized aching is compatible with either tonsillitis or an enterovirus 'flu-like illness (Echo or Coxsackie virus). Again, the only way to diagnose the presence of tonsillitis is to look at the throat.

In both adults and children there may be an associated cold-in-the-nose and/or cough. Roughly 40% of patients with streptococcal tonsillitis have these respiratory symptoms, and in non-streptococcal tonsillitis the incidence is a little higher at about 60%. This means that a full 'flu picture in the adult of pyrexia, headache, aching, cold, cough and sore throat (symptom), or a similar illness in children with vomiting instead of aching, could again represent either tonsillitis or a simple respiratory illness or a respiratory 'flu-like illness, and yet again, the only way to determine which, is to look at the throat.

Some patients with tonsillitis do not have a sore throat; a few will present as PUO, and some will have a thick voice as distinct from the husky voice of laryngitis.

Associated Illness Features

In addition to the cold and cough already described, a child may have delirium on the first night of the illness, or an adult a rigor, and rarely meningism may occur. Vomiting is commonest in children, but does occur in adults, and both may have diarrhoea. Non-specific abdominal pain commonly occurs in children. Other features of a respiratory illness sometimes occur and should be looked for or noted, e.g. otitis media, sinusitis, conjunctivitis, laryngitis, and it is even possible for tonsillitis and pneumonia to co-exist. Tonsillitis may cause referred ear pain in the absence of ear infection.

The Throat and Cervical Nodes

The inflamed tonsil varies from being red and swollen, to being grossly inflamed with overlying exudate or pus. In mild infection, absence of the surface blood vessels and loss of the crypt corrugations owing to oedema serve to diagnose inflammation. It may seem excessive to advocate a proper look at the throat, but the tonsils often extend much lower down behind the tongue than expected, and tongue depression is advisable unless the whole tonsillar bed is obviously visible. A partial view of the upper part of the tonsils can sometimes give an erroneous impression of normality, while in fact large and inflamed tonsils may be present but out of sight.

Tonsillar nodes may or may not be enlarged, and sometimes, despite the absence of node enlargement, there may be tenderness at the tonsillar node sites.

Treatment is discussed subsequently.

Scarlet Fever

The rash of scarlet fever represents infection with an erythrogenic strain of the β-haemolytic streptococcus in a person lacking immunity to the erythrogenic strain, but the illness is otherwise no different from other instances of tonsillitis.

Quinsy

The peritonsillar abscess is a formation of pus between the constrictor muscles and the lateral border of the tonsil. Clinically the patient is very ill, has a very painful throat, exhibits trismus and drools saliva owing to an inability to swallow. The tonsil is inflamed and pushed medially; the soft palate on the same side bulges downwards and forwards, and the uvula is displaced to the opposite side.

The β-haemolytic streptococcus is widely stated to be the cause, but Drake-Lee and Webber (1983) comment that the bacteriology of quinsies has not been well studied; that sometimes no organism is identified, and that an anaerobic streptococcus might sometimes have a causative role. The patient needs immediate hospital admission.

Conclusions

It is evident that tonsillitis is not an isolated disorder, but is very much part of a wider illness complex, and that viruses would seem to be implicated in causation. It is also evident that patients are often ill.

Other causes of tonsillitis or true pharyngitis are collectively much less common:

Glandular Fever

There may be no distinctive features between anginose glandular fever and 'ordinary' tonsillitis, but diagnostic suspicion would arise if the patient fails to respond quickly to antibiotics; if the patient is a teenager, or if there is redness of the soft palate and adjacent hard palate. Typically in glandular fever, the tonsillar nodes are larger (3 cm), often multinodular, and extend backwards beneath the upper end of the sternomastoid muscle.

Measles

Tonsillitis may occur during the prodromal phase, and is recognized usually in the older child. It is taken to represent an ordinary streptococcal or non-streptococcal tonsillitis because at this stage of the illness the clinical features are pyrexia, cold and cough.

Diphtheria

Sporadic cases still occur, but many general practitioners have never seen the disease, and while herd immunity persists, hopefully never will. It is helpful for those doctors who have never seen diphtheria to know that the diphtheritic membrane is very similar to the membranous slough seen a few days after tonsillectomy.

Candida

Seen usually in the elderly, often in the debilitated, and sometimes following antibiotics, the whole pharynx and palate are abnormally reddened and painful, but there is no oedema. The appearance is quite different from the white coating of 'thrush' seen in infants. Treatment by mouthwash of nystatin suspension is effective within 24–48 hours.

Gonococcal Pharyngitis

Oropharyngeal gonorrhoea is uncommon and may be asymptomatic. If the patient has a story of oro-genital contact the diagnosis is presumed and confirmed by swab and culture (Adler 1983). Antibiotic treatment encompasses the patient as a whole and specialist advice is advisable.

Pharyngeal Ulcers

Herpes simplex and Coxsackie viruses are the commonest causes, the clinical syndromes varying from the occasional ulcer to the ill child with a 'mouthful' of painful ulcers. The aphthous ulcer is described as a separate entity of uncertain cause. The vesicles of chicken pox will often involve the pharynx, and rarely herpes zoster will produce vesicles in the distribution of the ninth and tenth cranial nerves. In hand, foot and mouth disease (Coxsackie virus) discrete ulcers (starting as vesicles) throughout the oral cavity are seen in conjunction with vesicles on the hands, feet and legs, but in practice the limb vesicles are commonly present alone.

In treatment the accessible ulcer can be helped by sitting a hydrocortisone pellet (Corlan) on the ulcer, or by the local use of Adcortyl-in-Orabase, and more widespread ulceration by local anaesthetic mouth wash comprising 0.1% lignocaine in normal saline. Kellow (1984) obtained value from local carbenoxolone, and oral acyclovir may be used for herpes simplex.

The classic Vincent's angina has probably never been seen by many general practitioners. The ulcerative gingivo-stomatitis with pyrexia and foul-smelling breath is believed caused by a spirochaete in conjunction with a fusiform bacillus, in a patient already unwell owing to malnutrition or concomitant infection. Treatment with cleansing mouth washes, penicillin and metronidazole is followed by dental referral.

Leukaemia

Tonsillo-pharyngitis may be one of the presenting features, and clinically the illness may be initially mistaken for glandular fever.

Tumour

Squamous-cell carcinoma can produce an ulcerative mass in the region of the tonsil, and lympho-sarcoma causes unilateral enlargement of the tonsil.

Lassa Fever

Lassa fever is an arenavirus infection transmitted by the *Mastomys natatensis* rat, and the patient will become ill within three weeks of leaving the rural areas of Nigeria, Liberia or Sierra Leone. Illness features are persisting pyrexia sometimes with rigors, proteinurea, and a degree of lethargy and prostration greater than expected. The associated pharyngitis is occasionally absent.

Viruses and Bacteria in Tonsillitis

An understanding of cause is not easy because throat swabs will sometimes isolate a bacterium, less often a virus, occasionally both, but often neither.

Viruses

The range of viruses associated with tonsillitis (inflamed throat) are herpes simplex, adenoviruses, enteroviruses (Echo and Coxsackie), para-influenza viruses, rhino-viruses, Influenza A and Influenza B. The recorded total incidence varies from 20% (Poole and Tobin 1973) to 37% (Moffet *et al.* 1968). The three viral groups most commonly found are herpes simplex, adenoviruses and enteroviruses. Influenza A is rarely identified. Herpes simplex is likely to be acting as a primary invader, because most patients do not have the cold sores on the lips, or the buccal ulcers which are a feature of recrudescence of latent infection.

Most of the identified viruses occur in patients with non-streptococcal tonsillitis, and the proportionally highest incidence of all occurs in those few non-streptococcal instances which have no response at all to penicillin and may therefore initially be considered glandular fever suspects. Viruses are identified in streptococcal tonsillitis, but the incidence is lower.

How do these facts relate to the known clinical picture? About 40% of patients with streptococcal and 60% with non-streptococcal tonsillitis have an associated cold and/or cough, indicating involvement of a respiratory virus in causation. This indication is in keeping with the range of viruses identified and is not minimized by their low incidence, because the pick-up rate for viruses is known to be low.

What of tonsillitis without cold or cough, comprising again both streptococcal and non-streptococcal infection? The enteroviruses are known to produce a 'flu-like illness without respiratory features, and the enteroviruses are one of the commoner viruses identified in tonsillitis, and in both adults and children tonsillitis will often present as a non-respiratory 'flu illness. It is therefore possible that the enteroviruses have a causative role in tonsillitis occurring without respiratory features.

Conclusion

Both streptococcal and non-streptococcal tonsillitis may well have a viral cause. Of necessity, therefore, streptococcal tonsillitis would have a combined viral and bacterial cause, and because streptococcal and non-streptococcal tonsillitis have the same clinical picture, it is suggestive that a similar combined causation applies also to non-streptococcal tonsillitis.

If all patients with tonsillitis do have a combined cause, then there should be evidence to show that a combined viral/bacterial cause is feasible, and also evidence of a bacterial component in non-streptococcal tonsillitis despite the absence of a bacterial isolation.

Combined Viral and Bacterial Infection

Loosli (1968) quotes numerous examples in animals of combined viral/bacterial infection, and it is well known that in man a primary viral infection of the respiratory tract facilitates secondary bacterial infection. Nichol and Cherry (1967) found a 35% incidence of multiple agents (viral/bacterial, viral/viral) in 69 children with respiratory illness including tonsillitis. Epidemiological evidence of a dual origin for tonsillitis comes from a study of acute rheumatism in approved schools, when Bates (1967) found that in many cases acute rheumatism was associated with an increase in the number of cases of 'upper respiratory infection' occurring in the school. The implication is that streptococcal tonsillitis could be triggered by a viral infection.

Further evidence comes from the clinical material seen in general practice. Presented with a patient who has a 'flu-like illness and tonsillitis, it is puzzling to know whether the 'flu is causing the tonsillitis, or whether the tonsillitis is causing the 'flu. The remarkable similarity in the clinical picture between the common 'flu illness without tonsillitis and the less common 'flu illness with tonsillitis is strongly suggestive that the tonsillitis is due to secondary bacterial infection on a viral cause. Also suggestive is the patient with tonsillitis who presents as PUO; the delay in development of the visibly inflamed throat could well be explained by secondary bacterial invasion.

A Bacterial Cause in Non-Streptococcal Tonsillitis?
Penicillin Response

Comparing placebo with either sulphonamide or penicillin, Chapple *et al.* (1956) reported 61% of patients with 'acute febrile sore throat' still ill on the third day compared to half that number in the antibiotic groups, and that this result applied to both streptococcal and non-streptococcal infection. The findings by Merenstein and Rogers (1974) were similar, and in a study of patients with inflamed throats and receiving antibiotics (Everett 1979b), recovery times were constant irrespective of prior illness duration in both streptococcal and non-streptococcal tonsillitis, implying response to antibiotic, but the actual recovery times for non-streptococcal tonsillitis were marginally slower than for streptococcal infection.

These findings indicate a response to penicillin, and therefore suggest a bacterial involvement in non-streptococcal tonsillitis.

Why Unidentified?

A throat swab is a swab of the tonsil surface, and during an attack of tonsillitis it is possible that causative bacteria in the tonsil are not picked up on the surface. A discrepancy in isolation rates between the tonsil core and the tonsil surface has been demonstrated (Brook *et al.* 1980, Reilly *et al.* 1981), and Osborne and Roydhouse (1976) have clearly shown that repeated bouts of infection progressively impair crypt drainage. It is therefore entirely conceivable that bacteria should sometimes fail to reach the tonsil surface during an episode of acute inflammation, and it might then be argued that the marginally slower penicillin response in non-streptococcal tonsillitis is due to that same poor drainage which prevents isolation of the bacterium.

Another Pathogen?

The implied penicillin response to non-streptococcal tonsillitis suggests that neither staphylococci nor anaerobic bacteria have a pathogenic role because the incidence of β-lactamase production in both groups of organisms is high (Brook *et al.* 1981, Reilly *et al.* 1981). *Haemophilus influenzae*, while looked on as a commensal, might become pathogenic (Juel-Jensen *et al.* 1967) but there is no proof.

An Unidentified β-haemolytic Streptococcus?

It can be argued that there *is* no other pathogen, and that non-streptococcal tonsillitis is also caused by the β-haemolytic streptococcus, unidentified and responding more slowly to penicillin owing to impaired crypt drainage. This would readily explain why streptococcal and non-streptococcal tonsillitis have the same clinical picture.

In patients with tonsillitis, Merenstein and Rogers (1974) found that double-swabbing yielded a 6.8% increase in the isolation rates of β-haemolytic streptococcus, as compared to the use of a single swab, and Mortimer (1971) reviewed the literature relating to throat swabs in patients with scarlet fever. In only two of ten cited studies was there a 100% isolation rate of β-haemolytic streptococci, and the lowest isolation rates being 68% and 69% respectively.

Conclusions

The simple tenet that 'some are streptococcal and the rest are viral' is no longer acceptable. Streptococcal tonsillitis is likely to be initiated by a viral trigger, the streptococcus acting as a secondary bacterial invader and being responsible for the visible inflammation.

In non-streptococcal tonsillitis, the virus may play a greater role in aetiology, but is probably still acting predominantly as a trigger, the visible inflammation again being caused by secondary bacterial invasion. There is no proof for the existence of an alternative bacterial pathogen, but there is some evidence that the responsible bacterium might be an unidentified β-haemolytic streptococcus.

At the top of the viral spectrum it is possible that the few instances of non-streptococcal tonsillitis with total absence of penicillin response (glandular fever suspects) may be purely viral in origin.

Antibiotic Use

Unreliability of Throat Swab

The particular significance of the suggested causation of tonsillitis is that throat-swabbing may be an unreliable method of detecting the β-haemolytic streptococcus. This implication cuts across decades of thought and practice, and generates the need for a complete re-orientation in thinking. Much time and energy has gone into studies designed to distinguish clinically between streptococcal tonsillitis and non-streptococcal tonsillitis (inflamed throats) and these studies continue to be done now, but it is very probable that this line of thought is wrong and the time and energy wasted because it is entirely possible that streptococcal and 'non-streptococcal' tonsillitis are the same disease.

Throat swabs will continue to be taken but no longer can a negative result be reliably concluded to exclude the β-haemolytic streptococcus. Mathiassen (1980) writes that 'General practitioners' diagnostic and therapeutic problems are not solved by microbiological methods, but by sufficient knowledge and clinical experience'.

Recognition of Streptococcal Infection

Clinical distinction between streptococcal and non-streptococcal tonsillitis is known to lack reliability, and doubt is now cast on the reliability of the throat swab. What is left? Encompassing the *whole field* of sore throat, the answer is the clinical distinction between the non-inflamed and the inflamed throat. This enables a distinction to be made between what is known to be viral (non-inflamed sore throat), and what is believed to be combined viral and bacterial (inflamed throat), and this distinction embraces the knowledge that the inflamed throat includes both streptococcal and 'non-streptococcal infection', and that some of the latter may be streptococcal as well.

On looking at the throat, there is no longer need to ask 'Is this bacterial or viral?', but instead, 'Is this inflamed or non-inflamed?' Caplan (1979) argues against the need for throat swab, and recommends antibiotic treatment if the patient is ill and has an inflamed throat, and when Howie (1983) states that he still treats 'tonsils with spots on them and the reddest of the pharyngitises', is he not looking at the throat and deciding whether or not it looks inflamed, irrespective of whether it is 'viral' or 'bacterial', and irrespective of whether it is 'streptococcal' or 'non-streptococcal'?

Antibiotic Policy

Antibiotics should either be prescribed for all patients with an inflamed throat or for none. To do otherwise would be illogical. To make the point in another way: if for whatever clinical reason some patients with an inflamed throat receive an antibiotic and others do not, then quite arbitrarily, some patients with streptococcal tonsillitis will receive an antibiotic and others will not. The decision to use an antibiotic for the inflamed throat is therefore a policy decision, and does not depend upon any particular clinical features in any particular illness.

The question now is whether the inflamed throat *justifies* antibiotic use.

Deciding Factors for Antibiotic Use

A decision may be based upon the following considerations:

(1) *Illness Severity* In the section describing clinical features, it has already been noted that patients with tonsillitis are often ill.

(2) *The β-haemolytic Streptococcus* Despite a natural waning in virulence over the past few decades, 'modern' strains of streptococcus are endowed with formidable invasive powers, and can kill, and can do so very rapidly (*British Medical Journal* Leader 1970). Other reports emphasizing the same point have continued to appear (British Medical Journal Epidemiological Report 1972, Cargill *et al.* 1978, British Medical Journal Epidemiological Report 1978, Goepel *et al.* 1980, Cruikshank *et al.* 1981).

(3) *Benefit from Antibiotic Use?* The classic trial (Brumfitt and Slater 1957) compared penicillin against non-specific therapy in 60 young adults with Group A streptococcal tonsillitis, and demonstrated a 24 hour reduction in the duration of symptoms in those treated, and a similar finding was shown by Chapple *et al.* (1956) and Merenstein and Rogers (1974).

(4) *The Untreated Course* Dr G.I. Watson (1982) has written 'Streptococcal pharyngitis may remain clinically mild for several days before subsiding for a while, but relapses are common and such a patient may remain infectious for three weeks or longer'.

(5) *Suppurative Complications* These include otitis media, sinusitis, quinsy, retropharyngeal abscess and suppurative cervical nodes, but the extent to which they might occur if antibiotics were widely withheld is not known.

Treatment Policy Decision

I would use an antibiotic for all patients with an inflamed throat because patients are often ill; because the β-haemolytic streptococcus is potentially dangerous, and because there is a 24 hour gain in clinical recovery. It is acknowledged that the cited instances of streptococcal ferocity occur rarely and are mostly unrelated to the throat, but in the context of respiratory illness as a whole, it seems foolhardy to withhold antibiotics from a minority group associated with a bacterium known to have this potential. Similarly, the 24 hour gain in clinical recovery may seem of little moment to an armchair discussion, but assumes a different significance in the eyes of the patient.

Antibiotic indication in the whole field of sore throat is summarized in Figure 4.2.

INFLAMED THROAT

Antibiotic Use

Tonsillitis		
Tonsillo-pharyngitis	Streptococcal and 'non-streptococcal'	YES
True pharyngitis		

NON-INFLAMED THROAT

Normal redness		NO
Quasi-pharyngitis		
Bypass phenomenon	*	YES
Recurrent tonsillitis		

Figure 4.2 Antibiotic indication in sore throat
* See text page 45

Antibiotic Choice and Treatment Duration

In choosing the best antibiotic it is necessary to distinguish between clinical recovery and eradication of the streptococcus. The comment that 'a growing number of children with tonsillitis become refractory to therapy with penicillin' (Brook *et al.* 1981) relates not to clinical recovery, but to eradication of the organism. The immediate objective is to aid swift clinical recovery, but should eradication also be an aim? Rheumatic fever prevention can no longer be considered a valid reason, but persistence of the organism in the throat following antibiotic treatment can lead to a relapse of clinical tonsillitis in a small proportion of patients. An attempt to eradicate the streptococcus could reduce this incidence.

The traditional method of eradication has been the ten day antibiotic course, but with the impetus of rheumatic fever prevention gone, and the problem of compliance ever present, this approach is no longer acceptable. In fact it is probable that a majority of general practitioners long ago settled for a shorter course, and the relapse rate after a five day course of treatment is only slightly higher than the relapse rate after ten days (Hansen *et al*. 1983). It may be possible, however, to achieve both clinical recovery and a degree of eradication by antibiotic choice.

Brook *et al*. (1981) have suggested that β-lactamase (penicillinase) producing staphylococci and anaerobic bacteria in the throat can limit the efficiency of penicillin therapy by enzymatically disarming the penicillin, allowing the infection to continue. The extent of this phenomenon cannot be great, but an ideal antibiotic choice might be an antibiotic effective against both the β-haemolytic streptococcus and β-lactamase producing organisms. As such either erythromycin or a cephalosporin combined with metronidazole could be an ideal. In reality, however, it is questionable whether two antibiotics instead of one are justified purely to reduce a relapse rate which is already low, and most doctors would reasonably continue to use either phenoxymethylpenicillin or erythromycin alone. The β-haemolytic streptococcus remains universally sensitive to penicillin, but erythromycin-resistant strains have been reported in Liverpool (Youngs 1984) and Cambridge (Walker *et al*. 1984) in an incidence of 0.3% and 2.6% respectively. Co-trimoxazole is not a good choice; there are problems with sensitivity testing (Bushby 1973), and it is not always clinically effective.

Glandular Fever

β-Haemolytic streptococci are sometimes isolated by throat swab and for this reason the use of an antibiotic is advisable. In order to avoid the 'ampicillin rash', ampicillin, amoxycillin, and augmentin are avoided in teenagers or if glandular fever is clinically suspect, but a majority of smaller children with tonsillitis do not have glandular fever, and these broader spectrum penicillins may be used instead of phenoxymethylpenicillin if an additional illness feature such as otitis media co-exists.

The combination of metronidazole with penicillin can shorten both the duration of the tonsillitis and the febrile period (Hedström 1980). The indication that cephalexin produces rapid resolution of symptoms in glandular fever (Lakie 1983) needs confirmation.

Measles

Because the tonsillitis occurs during the prodromal phase, the true diagnosis may not be apparent, and the patient will be treated as though having streptococcal/non-streptococcal infection.

Illness Management

There is variation in the speed of recovery, but most patients are appreciably better after 48 hours' antibiotic treatment. It is therefore convenient to advise a patient to return in 48 hours if not better. Failure to improve after three or four days indicates glandular fever or a viral infection mimicking glandular fever.

The usual method used for diagnosing glandular fever is to demonstrate the presence of heterophil antibody (Paul Bunnell, Monospot), but about 15% of patients with glandular fever are heterophil antibody negative. The diagnosis can be made with greater certainty by demonstrating the presence of Epstein Barr specific IgM. The possibility of an alternative viral infection might be clarified by viral throat swab and/or complement fixation tests performed on paired sera.

The Very Sore Throat

In the absence of quinsy, a patient with tonsillitis will rarely have so much pain in the throat that he is barely able to swallow his own saliva. The diagnosis may be glandular fever. If home management is unacceptable, then intravenous fluid and antibiotic in hospital becomes necessary.

Prophylaxis

A single 125 mg daily dose of penicillin is effective in reducing the number of attacks of tonsillitis in children with recurrent tonsillitis (Donovan 1973). Because prophylaxis is neither a substitute for, nor as effective as tonsillectomy, it is best used for children on the waiting list for tonsillectomy.

REFERRAL FOR TONSILLECTOMY

Tonsillectomy, as distinct from adenoidectomy, may be necessary in the following situations.

Recurrent Tonsillitis

Referral is justified if the child is having three or more objectively recorded attacks of tonsillitis a year. By keeping an objective record the general practitioner can be of help to the ENT surgeon, who has only the mother's story and the tonsil appearance to guide him. The mother's story is an unreliable means of diagnosing tonsillitis, and the tonsil appearance alone may be inadequate.

Immunological memory and the child's subsequent ability to respond to infection are unaltered by tonsillectomy (Veltri *et al.* 1972), but the higher incidence of meningococcal carriers following tonsillectomy (Kristiansen *et al.* 1984) suggests that some impairment of immune mechanisms might occur.

Adult referral is made less often, and is justified after one or two bad attacks.

Tonsil Size

Obstruction resulting in snoring, sleep apnoea and possibly cor pulmonale is more likely to be caused by enlarged adenoids, but large tonsils may sometimes be responsible.

Quinsy

The patient will have been admitted as an emergency, and tonsillectomy is usually performed after subsidence of the acute inflammation.

REFERENCES

Adler, M. W. (1983). Complications of common genital infections and infections in other sites. *Br. Med. J.*, **287**, 1709–1712

Bates, M. M. (1967). Acute rheumatism in approved schools in England and Wales 1960–65. *Mon. Bull. Minist. Health Public Health Lab. Serv.*, **26**, 132–142

Bridges-Webb, C. (1977). Acute pharyngitis, tonsillitis and tonsillectomy. *Aust. Fam. Physician*, **6**, 498–509

British Medical Journal (1970). Leading Article 'Streptococcal sepsis'. **1**, 513–514

British Medical Journal (1972). Epidemiological Report '*Streptococcus pyogenes* deaths'. **4**, 437

British Medical Journal (1978). Epidemiological Report 'Bacteriaemia due to group A streptococci'. **1**, 1153

Brook, I., Yocum, P. and Shah, K. (1980). Surface vs. core-tonsillar aerobic and anaerobic flora in recurrent tonsillitis. *J. Am. Med. Assoc.*, **244**, 1696–1698

Brook, I., Yocum, P. and Friedman, E. M. (1981). Aerobic and anaerobic bacteria in tonsils of children with recurrent tonsillitis. *Ann. Otol. Rhinol. Laryngol.*, **90**, 261–263

Brumfitt, W. and Slater, J. D. H. (1957). Treatment of acute sore throat with penicillin. A controlled trial in young soldiers. *Lancet*, **1**, 8–11

Bushby, S. R. M. (1973). Sensitivity testing with trimethoprim/sulphamethoxazole. *Med. J. Aust. Special Supplement*, **1**, 10–18

Caplan, C. (1979). A case against the use of the throat culture in the management of streptococcal pharyngitis. *J. Fam. Pract.*, **8**, 485–490

Cargill, J. S., Harry, D. S. and Hutchinson, G. (1978). Diarrhoea – a cautionary tale. *The Practitioner*, **221**, 117–119

Chapple, P. A. L., Franklin, L. M., Paulett, J. D., Tuckman, E., Woodall, J. T., Tomlinson, A. J. H. and McDonald, J. C. (1956). The treatment of acute sore throat in general practice. Therapeutic trial, with observations on symptoms and bacteriology. *Br. Med. J.*, **1**, 705–708

Combined Study by the East Scotland Faculty, Royal College of General Practitioners, and the Department of Bacteriology, The University, Dundee (1975). Acute sore throat – Diagnosis and treatment in general practice. *J. R. Coll. Gen. Pract.*, **25**, 126–132

Cruikshank, J. G., Hart, R. C. J., George, M. and Feest, T. G. (1981). Fatal streptococcal septicaemia. *Br. Med. J.*, **282**, 1944–1945

Donovan, R. (1973). Clinical and immunological studies on children undergoing tonsillectomy for repeated sore throats. *Proc. R. Soc. Med. (Sect. Laryngol.)*, **66**, 413–416

Drake-Lee, A. B. and Webber, P. A. (1983). Adenotonsillectomy: current debate. *The Practitioner*, **227**, 929–933

Evans, C. E., McFarlane, A. H., Norman, G. R., Neale, K. A. and Streiner, D. L. (1982). *Can. Fam. Physician*, **28**, 453–458

Everett, M. T. (1979a). The uninflamed sore throat. *The Practitioner*, **222**, 835–838

Everett, M. T. (1979b). The cause of tonsillitis. *The Practitioner*, **223**, 253–259

Feery, B. J., Forsell, P. and Gulasekharam, J. (1976). Streptococcal sore throat in general practice – a controlled study. *Med. J. Aust.*, **1**, 989–991

Goepel, J. R., Richards, D. G., Harris, D. M. and Henry, L. (1980). Fulminant *Streptococcus pyogenes* infection. *Br. Med. J.*, **281**, 1412

Griffiths, E. (1979). Incidence of ENT problems in general practice. *J. R. Soc. Med.*, **72**, 740–742

Hansen, J. G., Schmidt, H. and Bitsch, N. (1983). Sore throat. Principles of diagnosis and treatment. *The Practitioner*, **227**, 937–948

Hedström, S. A. (1980). Treatment of anginose infectious mononucleosis with metronidazole. *Scand. J. Infect. Dis.*, **12**, 265–269

Howie, J. G. R. (1983). Penicillin for sore throats (Letter to Editor). *The Practitioner*, **227**, 1349

Juel-Jensen, B. E., MacCullum, F. O. and Smith, J. W. G. (1967). Sore Throats. A combined clinical and laboratory study. *Proc. Br. Student Health (Officers) Assoc.*, **27**, 27–39

Kellow, J. E. (1984). Topical carbenoxalone therapy for acute stomatitis. *Med. J. Aust.*, **141**, 40

Kristiansen, B.-E., Elverland, H. and Hannestad, K. (1984). Increased meningococcal carrier rate after tonsillectomy. *Br. Med. J.*, **288**, 974

Lakie, J. (1983). Use of cephalexin to treat glandular fever: pilot study. *Br. Med. J.*, **286**, 1617–1618

Loosli, C. G. (1968). Synergism between respiratory virus and bacteria. *Yale J. Biol. Med.*, **40**, 522–539

Mathiassen, P. (1980). Sore throats and microbiological diagnosis. *Ugeskr. Laeg.*, **142**, 511–512

Merenstein, J. H. and Rogers, K. D. (1974). Streptococcal pharyngitis. *J. Am. Med. Assoc.*, **227**, 1278–1282

Moffett, H. L., Siegal, A. C. and Doyle, H. K. (1968). Non-streptococcal pharyngitis. *J. Pediatr.*, **73**, 51–60

Mortimer, E. A. (1971). Rheumatic fever, throat cultures, and penicillin. *Paediatrics*, **48**, 843–845

Nichol, K. P. and Cherry, J. D. (1967). Bacterial-viral interrelations in respiratory infections of children. *New Engl. J. Med.*, **277**, 667–672

Osborne, G. R. and Roydhouse, N. (1976). The Tonsillitis Habit, (Auckland, New Zealand: W. P. Roydhouse)

Poole, P. M. and Tobin, J. O'H. (1973). Viral and epidemiological findings in MRC/PHLS surveys of respiratory disease in hospital and general practice. *Postgrad. Med. J.*, **49**, 778–787

Reilly, S., Timmis, P., Beeden, A. G. and Willis, A. T. (1981). Possible role of the anaerobe in tonsillitis. *J. Clin. Path.*, **34**, 542–547

Shaheen, O. H. (1983). Managing the causes of sore throat. *Mod. Med.*, **28**, No. 2, 48–51

Valkenberg, H. A., Haverkorn, M. J., Goslings, W. R. O., Lorrier, J. C., de Moor, C. E. and Maxted, W. R. (1971). The attack rate of rheumatic fever and acute glomerulonephritis in patients not treated with penicillin. *J. Infect. Dis.*, **124**, 348–358

Veltri, R. W., Sprinkle, P. M., Keller, S. A. and Chicklo, J. M. (1972). Immunoglobulin changes in a pediatric otolaryngic patient sample subsequent to T. & A. *J. Laryngol. Otol.*, **86**, 905–916

Walker, M., Whetstone, R. J. and Whipp, J. (1984). Erythromycin resistant *Streptococcus pyogenes* in Cambridge. *J. Infect.*, **8**, 88–89

Watson, G. I. (1982). *Epidemiology and Research in a General Practice*. The Royal College of General Practitioners

Youngs, E. R. (1984). Erythromycin resistant *Streptococcus pyogenes* in Merseyside. *J. Infect.*, **8**, 86–87

5
Otitis Media

Use of the Auroscope – Clinical Features of Acute Otitis Media – Bacteria in Acute Otitis Media – Secretory Otitis Media – Management and Antibiotic Use – Chronic Otitis Media

USE OF THE AUROSCOPE

The mother sits facing the doctor, with the child sitting sideways on his mother's lap, resting his head against her chest. One of the mother's hands holds the child's head, and the other restrains the child's free arm which might otherwise wipe the auroscope away. In Figure 5.1 the position of the mother's hands is incorrect, because the child's vision is obscured and will cause restlessness. The correct position is demonstrated in Figure 5.2.

The technique depicted in Figure 5.3 is wrong because the doctor's hand and the child's head are two separate entities. If the child suddenly moves his head despite the mother's restraining hand, the auroscope could damage the external auditory meatus. A correct technique is depicted in Figure 5.4. The doctor should kneel so that his eye is on a level with the child's head, and one hand gently pulls the ear backwards. The other hand holds the auroscope in an underarm position, which enables the free fingers of that hand to rest against the child's cheek. In this way the doctor's operative hand, the auroscope and the child's head become one entity, and any unexpected movements of the child's head are transmitted to the auroscope. Figure 5.5 is the same as Figure 5.4 but is viewed from beneath to show the fingers resting on the face.

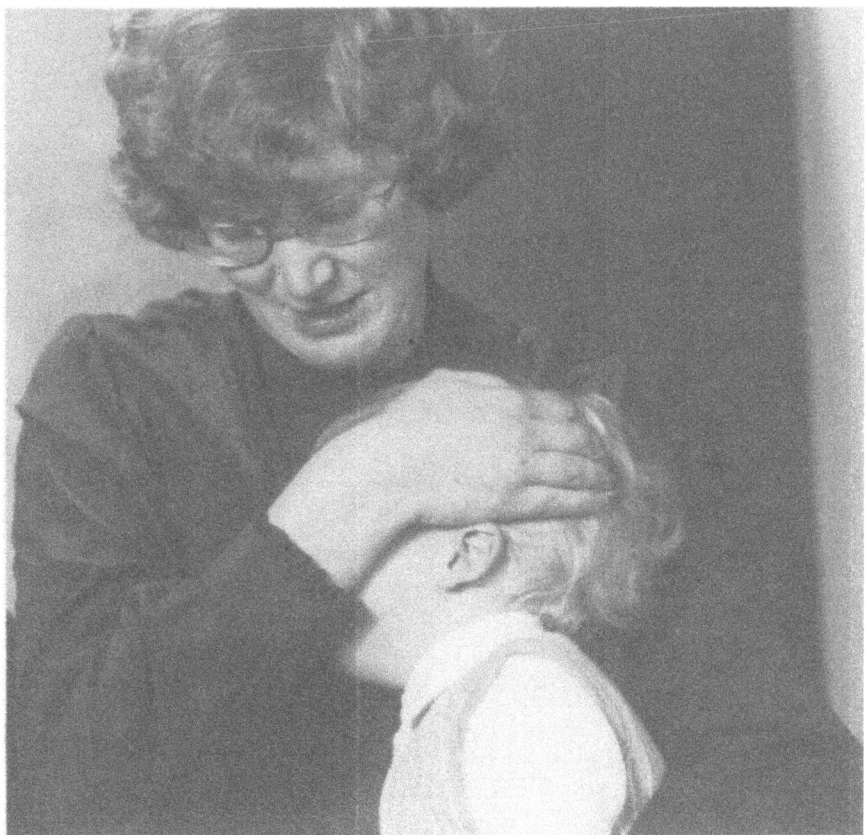

Figure 5.1 Incorrect use of mother's hands

CLINICAL FEATURES OF ACUTE OTITIS MEDIA

Acute otitis media is most common in children under five years of age, and is seen less often in older children and adults. Otitis media can appear as an isolated disorder but is much more often associated with a respiratory viral infection. The whole range of respiratory viruses have been identified in association with the respiratory illnesses of which otitis media forms a part; rhinoviruses, adenoviruses, respiratory syncytial virus, parainfluenza viruses, Influenza A, Influenza B, and herpes simplex (Poole and Tobin 1973). Otitis media is also common in measles and in rotavirus infections.

Earache is common in those old enough to complain of pain, but may sometimes be absent, and the younger child can only cry or be restless. A young child will typically have a cold with perhaps a cough, and may then develop a temperature and/or crying. Other symptoms

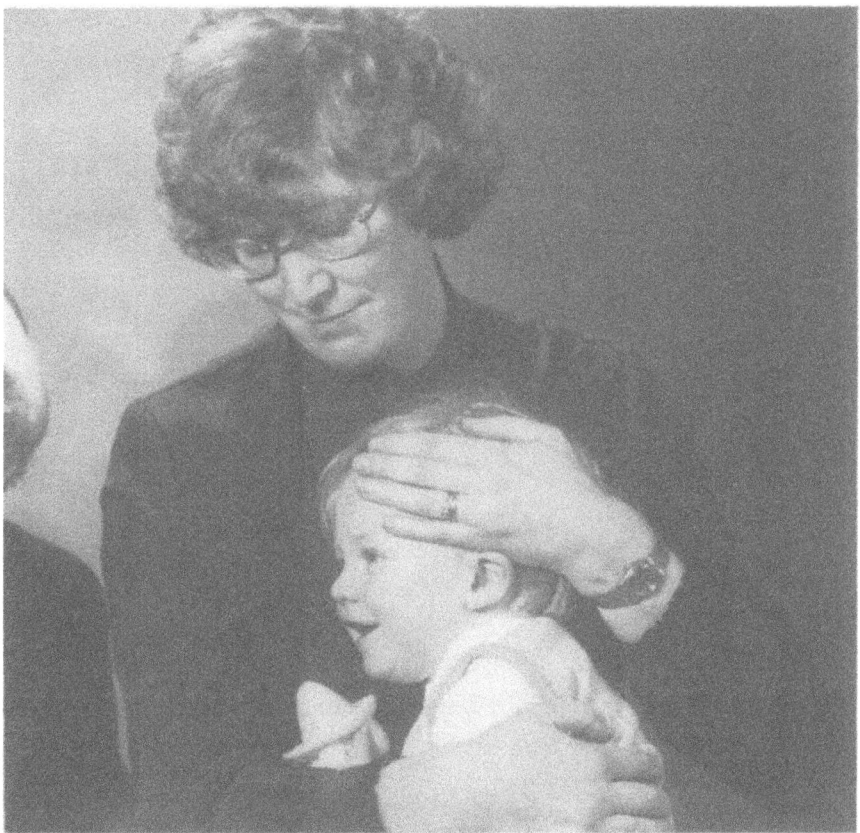

Figure 2 Correct position of mother's hands

include non-specific vomiting and less often diarrhoea. Otitis media can also present as PUO.

The Inflamed Drum

Hyperaemia

Blood vessels on the drum give it an 'injected' appearance which does not indicate frank otitis media but may represent an early stage.

Redness

A part or whole of the drum is obviously red, and this is the finding most often seen.

68 Selective Antibiotic Use in Respiratory Illness

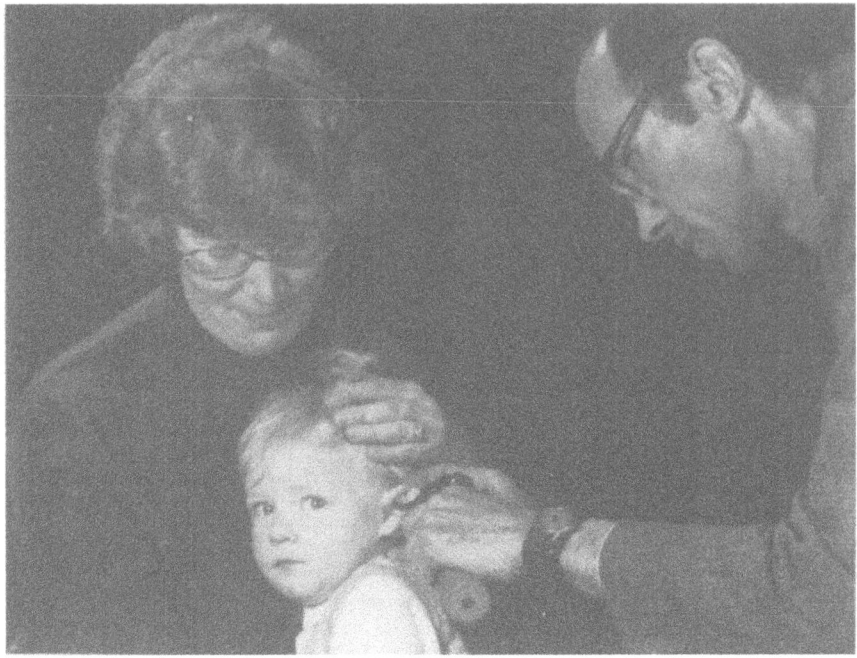

Figure 5.3 Incorrect technique when using an auroscope

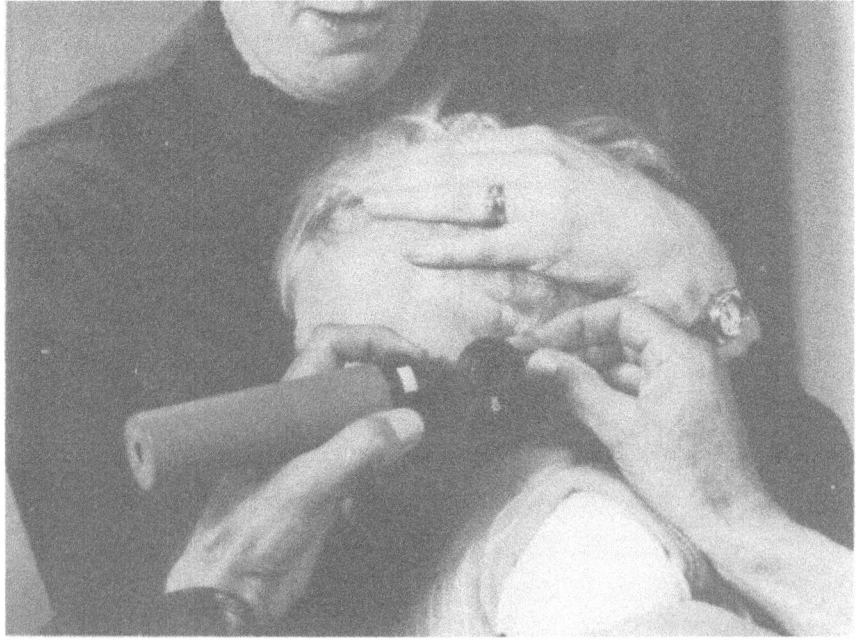

Figure 5.4 A correct technique when using an auroscope

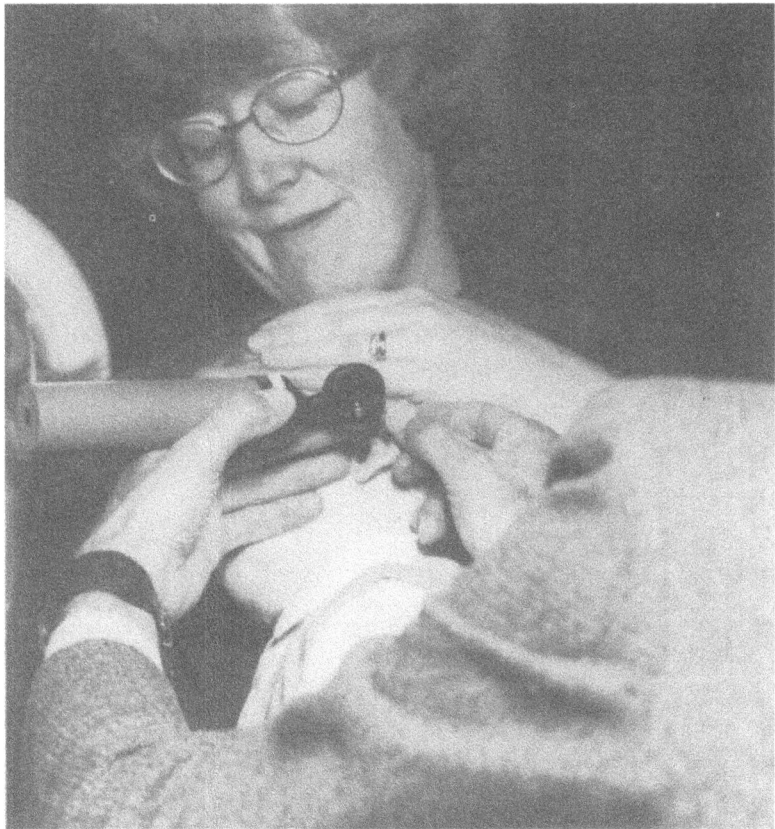

Figure 5.5 A correct technique depicting contact of doctor's hand with child's face

Granular Appearance

The entire drum is covered by multiple greyish-white 'cobblestones' set on a dull red background. The 'cobblestones' are 1–2 mm in size as viewed through the auroscope. This variety of acute otitis media is not uncommon yet is seemingly undescribed, and its distinctive appearance suggests a specific infective cause, but both clinical features and antibiotic response are the same as in children with a red drum.

Bullae

Pinkish bullae are quite common. Haemorrhagic bullae are seen much less often and are attributed to *Mycoplasma pneumoniae*, but have been seen also in an adult with Influenza B infection.

Perforation

If perforation of the drum occurs, the pain disappears and the external auditory meatus becomes filled with pus. A view of the drum is obviously impossible and there is no requirement to mop out the pus in order to see it.

Haemorrhage

Bleeding from the ear is rare in acute otitis media, but can occur in association with the discharge if the drum perforates. Grace et al. (1984) caution that recurrent bleeding from the ear is likely to be caused by non-accidental injury.

Obscuration by Wax

When the drum is obscured by wax, both diagnosis and treatment have to be based upon presumption.

Differential Diagnosis of Earache

The teeth, the throat and the neck are the three common areas to check. Tonsillitis commonly causes referred ear pain, and dental causes are well-known. In adults of a relevant age, cervical spondylosis may cause pain in the region of the ear. Other causes include a furuncle in the external auditory meatus, mumps and, rarely, herpes zoster oticus (Ramsay Hunt syndrome) seen usually in the elderly. Sometimes *secretory* otitis media causes transient earache.

Recurrent Otitis Media

Thought should be given to the possibility of adenoidal hyperplasia and associated sinus infection, but the finding by Branefors-Helander et al. (1975) that different bacterial species or serotypes were usually isolated in successive episodes of acute otitis media suggests that recurring attacks reflect the propensity of small children to contract recurring viral infections, which in turn lead to otitis media.

Complications

Acute mastoiditis and meningitis are possible but are now rare. Untreated or inappropriately treated acute otitis media can result in chronic otitis media.

Secretory Otitis Media and Deafness

Shurin *et al.* (1979) found a persistent middle ear effusion in 42% of 107 children checked between two and thirteen weeks after acute otitis media, and the incidence was highest in those under the age of two years. More recently, Barritt and Darbyshire (1984) similarly recorded an incidence of secretory otitis media and deafness following acute otitis media.

BACTERIA IN ACUTE OTITIS MEDIA

Bacteriological assessment of acute otitis media by tympanocentesis has produced uniform results in many studies. Pathogenic bacteria are isolated in two thirds of patients, and *Streptococcus pneumoniae* and *Haemophilus influenzae* are the two common infective agents, sometimes occurring together. β-Haemolytic streptococci and *Staphylococcus aureus* are infrequent causes. It is perhaps less well appreciated that *H. influenzae* is as common over the age of five years, as under (Howie *et al.* 1970, Schwartz *et al.* 1977, Schwartz and Rodriguez 1981).

No Bacterial Pathogen

In one third of patients with acute otitis media, no bacterial pathogen is identified. It is easy to presume that the cause in these instances is viral, but there is no certainty that this presumption is right. Viruses are rarely identified in middle ear fluid obtained by tympanocentesis (Halsted *et al.* 1968, Klein and Teele 1976), and although their absence does not necessarily exclude a viral cause, it would seem much more likely that most instances of acute otitis media represent a secondary bacterial infection on a viral trigger. If this is so, what is the nature of the unidentified bacterium? One possibility is anaerobic bacteria, which were identified by tympanocentesis in 63.4% of 186 children with acute otitis media (Brook 1979). Another possibility is that host mechanisms may have already eliminated pathogenic bacteria by the time tympanocentesis is performed (Rowe 1975).

Rare Causes

Gram-negative enteric bacilli, and *Chlamydia trachomatis* are rare causes in infants, and *M. pneumoniae* is a rare cause in any age group. In the immuno-compromised patient, the bacteriological possibilities are wide.

SECRETORY OTITIS MEDIA

Secretory otitis media (serous otitis media, glue-ear, middle ear effusion) is discussed now, 'in the middle of acute otitis media' as it were, because an understanding of secretory otitis media has possible relevance to antibiotic use in *acute* otitis media.

Secretory otitis media is the commonest cause of deafness in children, and is now well-recognized in small children as well as in the older 5–8 year age range. The clinical presentation may include recurrent attacks of acute otitis media, but relates primarily to poor hearing. This can be detected from a very early age by hearing tests, and if unrecognized becomes manifest clinically as delay or abnormality in speech development, poor learning and/or bad behaviour. The middle ear cavity contains fluid which may attain a glue-like consistency, and the drum appears dull and yellow without a light reflex, and may be hyperaemic with visible blood vessels. Later, the handle of the malleus retracts inwards and the lateral process becomes prominent, and fluid levels may be seen.

Cause

The cause is problematical. For some reason the fluid cannot drain along the Eustachian tube. Because secretory otitis media is usually bilateral, a central cause is implied, and adenoidal hyperplasia undoubtedly contributes to causation. Sinusitis and the more common allergic rhinitis are also contributory factors. Some, but not all instances, follow acute otitis media (Shurin *et al.* 1979, Barritt and Darbyshire 1984).

The Role of Antibiotics

Secretory otitis media achieved greater recognition after the advent of antibiotic use for acute otitis media, and such use has been implicated as a cause. Lim *et al.* (1980) argue that if secretory otitis media is caused by inappropriate or incomplete antibiotic treatment of acute otitis media, then there should be evidence of bacterial resistance in the middle ear fluid. Among a wide range of bacteria isolated from 82 of 182 ears in children with secretory otitis media aged between one and 11 years, these authors found that almost half the *H. influenzae* isolations were resistant to ampicillin, and suggest that incomplete or inappropriate antibiotic use in acute otitis media could select for antibiotic-resistant strains of bacteria, allowing prolonged irritation of the middle ear mucosa by bacteria not destroyed by the suboptimal levels of antibiotic.

These findings do *not* necessarily mean that antibiotics should be withheld in patients with acute otitis media, but they *could* mean that care should be taken in antibiotic choice, and thought given to antibiotic duration. These points, and the management of secretory otitis media itself, are discussed subsequently.

MANAGEMENT AND ANTIBIOTIC USE

Antibiotic Need in Acute Otitis Media

Should antibiotics be used in the treatment of acute otitis media? The easy answer is 'yes' because two thirds have a proven bacterial cause, and because the incidence of suppurative complications has declined since the advent of antibiotic use, but there is also evidence to show that many patients recover spontaneously without antibiotics. Antibiotics can relieve pain; in a trial of penicillin versus placebo in 150 children aged one to 10 years (Mygind *et al.* 1981), pain relief was significantly faster (after one or two doses) in those with a *Str. pneumoniae* isolation, whereas this effect was not apparent in those with *H. influenzae*. This discrepancy is no surprise because penicillin is not very active against *H. influenzae*. Might a more widespread relief of pain have been effected by use of a more appropriate antibiotic?

Conclusions

I shall continue to use antibiotics for the treatment of acute otitis media (except possibly in children with injected drums only) for the following reasons:

(1) Although some patients can recover spontaneously, others *do* need antibiotics, and it may not be easy, in advance, to distinguish one group from the other.

(2) It seems wrong to wait until the patient is worse before prescribing an antibiotic. It seems wrong to wait, for example, until a drum perforates, and it seems wrong to wait, as suggested by van Buchem *et al.* (1981), until the ear has discharged for two weeks before using an antibiotic. Rapid resolution of infection without perforation should be the ideal, and if perforated, the quicker the healing the better. The *existence* of a perforation is one step nearer to the possibility of chronic otitis media, and a prolonged discharge enchances this possibility.

(3) Trial evidence that pain is quickly relieved by an antibiotic is borne out by experience. It seems wrong to withhold an antibiotic knowing that its use could be more effective than simple analgesia.

(4) The fourth reason relates to respiratory illness as a whole. The point has already been made in Chapter 2 that it could be less relevant to make too big an issue about withholding antibiotics, in smaller groups of patients who do have a bacterial cause. In the whole field of respiratory illness, a selective antibiotic policy *does* withhold antibiotics from a larger number of patients with uncomplicated colds, coughs, 'flu-like illnesses and influenza, and the advice against antibiotic use in these instances can be given with sincerity because the illnesses are of viral origin and will not benefit. The execution of this selective antibiotic policy could lose credibility if antibiotics were withheld also from patients with acute otitis media.

Antibiotic Choice in Acute Otitis Media
Penicillin and Erythromycin

It needs to be emphasized that neither penicillin nor erythromycin are ideal. Both are effective against *Streptococcus pneumoniae*, but are less active against *H. influenzae* (Howie and Ploussard 1972, Howard *et al.* 1976). The implied recommendation in the British National Formulary (1984) that penicillin may be given if a patient is over the age of five years is wrong. The recommendation is based upon the belief that *H. influenzae* is confined to young children only, but this is not so.

Amoxycillin

Amoxycillin is widely used and is nearly always effective, but there are now two reasons why it might not be the best first choice:

(1) The occasional clinical treatment failure with amoxycillin reflects the known 6.6% incidence of *H. influenzae* resistance to ampicillin (Philpott-Howard and Williams 1982), and in such instances the use of co-trimoxazole or cefaclor, or sometimes augmentin, will effect cure. The incidence of such clinical failures is small and probably does not in itself constitute adequate reason for the abandonment of amoxycillin as a first choice, but as already mentioned:

(2) The suggestion by Lim *et al.* (1980) that inappropriate antibiotic choice might cause secretory otitis media, implies that *because* there is a 6.6% incidence of *H. influenzae* resistance to ampicillin (and amoxycillin), then neither ampicillin nor amoxycillin are the best choices. A trial, for example, comparing cefaclor with amoxycillin, would clarify whether the incidence of secretory otitis media is lower following the use of cefaclor. Such a trial (John and Vallé-Jones 1983) did not include a record of longer-term follow-up, but in the short-term those treated with cefaclor showed a greater number of tympanic membranes returning to their normal appearance, and a greater resolution of deafness. Both these findings imply that the incidence of secretory otitis media would be lower.

Augmentin

Clavulanate-potentiated amoxycillin would at first sight seem to be one answer to *H. influenzae* resistance. Although the incidence of resistance is relatively low (6.6%), the incidence of *H. influenzae* as a cause of acute otitis media is quite high, and the gain of augmentin over amoxycillin should therefore be measurable. In fact, however, only half the resistant strains of *H. influenzae* are resistant by virtue of β-lactamase production (Bell and Plowman 1980), and the gain of augmentin over amoxycillin would relate to this half only.

Cefaclor and Co-trimoxazole

These antibiotics are active against both *Str. pneumoniae* and *H. influenzae*, and would at present seem to be the best choice for the treatment of acute otitis media, when used in conventional dosage and for a conventional duration (see below).

Metronidazole

Specific treatment for the possibility of anaerobic bacteria in acute otitis media is not necessary because these bacteria have a relatively low pathogenicity and are likely to be adequately controlled by the antibiotic in use for the aerobic infection.

Antibiotic Duration in Acute Otitis Media

To know that a five day course of penicillin is as effective as a 10 day course (Ingvarrson and Lundgren 1982) is superficially of little moment because few general practitioners would now give more than a five day course, but in fact, this finding is of some significance because the authors also demonstrated that the incidence of subsequent secretory otitis media was not increased by the shorter course.

Owing to the usually rapid resolution of acute otitis media, interest is now focused on whether an even shorter course would be effective and safe. Two and three day courses are indeed effective (Chaput de Saintonge *et al.* 1982, Meistrup-Larsen *et al.* 1983), but the particular question is whether a two or three day antibiotic course will result in a higher incidence of secretory otitis media. As already discussed, the occurrence of secretory otitis media following acute otitis media might have its origin in a persistence of bacteria in the middle ear cavity, and it is conceivable that a very short antibiotic course, irrespective of antibiotic choice, might allow a bacterial persistence despite clinical recovery. Bain *et al.* (1985) have now demonstrated that high dose amoxycillin (750 mg twice daily) given for two days to children with acute otitis media aged three days and over is as effective as a conventional one week course in resolving symptoms and signs, and in particular resulted in no difference in the incidence of recurrent otitis media up to twelve months follow-up, or in hearing loss recorded at one month and six months after treatment. These results imply that a short course of amoxycillin in the dosage stated does not cause an increased incidence of secretory otitis media.

Other Treatments in Acute Otitis Media

Oral decongestants and antihistamines confer no therapeutic benefit and are responsible for an incidence of side effects (Bain 1983). Ear drops of any kind should not be used if the drum is perforated because several topical agents, e.g. neomycin, gentamicin, polymyxin B, can cause deafness by direct toxic effect. Antibiotic drops are ineffective in acute otitis media, but analgesic drops, e.g. choline salicylate with ethylene oxide-polyoxypropyleneglycol (Audax) can be beneficial and may be used if the drum is intact.

Illness Management

Acute Otitis Media

The Acute Illness

Should children with earache be visited during the night? The answer is preferably 'yes' because a single starter dose of antibiotic from the doctor's bag is likely to achieve faster pain relief than simple analgesia. A possible alternative is to provide analgesic eardrops in reserve, with the instruction to make an appointment the next morning if they are used, but this approach is not ideal; the mother will be less motivated to attend the surgery if pain is eased, and an untreated inflamed ear could progress to perforation.

In children with a perforated drum the ear should be allowed to drain freely, and the mother is advised not to plug the meatus except temporarily, for example, during bathing or hair-washing. The child is seen again definitively after the antibiotic course in order to confirm healing of the drum.

The Longer-Term

Longer-term management concerns recognition of deafness caused by secretory otitis media. Acknowledging the difficulties related to definitive hearing tests, particularly in young children, Barritt and Darbyshire (1984) found the appearance of the eardrum to be an accurate predictor of deafness, and the authors felt that a general practitioner would recognize an abnormal drum even if the exact abnormalities could not be specified. Based upon their findings, the authors suggest that a child should be seen six weeks after the acute episode of otitis media, and if the drum is abnormal, then audiometry should be undertaken after a further six weeks. By this time, half of those with abnormal drums will have regained hearing spontaneously, but the other half will remain deaf and require referral.

Secretory Otitis Media

Prevention

The use of oral decongestants during the treatment of *acute* otitis media did not prevent the subsequent development of secretory otitis media (Barritt and Darbyshire 1984), but argument has been presented for the possible preventive effects of appropriate antibiotic choice when treating acute otitis media.

Treatment

The essence of treatment is adenoidectomy, myringotomy, removal of the 'glue' by suction, and the insertion of grommets. There is current controversy about the need for surgical treatment, with the expressed viewpoint that operative treatment is undertaken too often and unnecessarily. While it is acknowledged that glue-ear will often resolve given time, e.g. three months, it has to be recognized that deafness is a major drawback to learning skills and speech development in a young child.

Neither oral decongestants nor decongestant-antihistamine combinations (Olsen *et al.* 1978, Cantekin *et al.* 1983) confer any benefit, but a month's use of the mucolytic carbocysteine (Mucodyne) gives modest benefit (Taylor and Dareshani 1975).

Prevention of Acute Otitis Media

Decongestants and antihistamines are ineffective in prevention (Randall and Hendley 1979, Bain 1983) and have no useful place in any sphere of otitis media (Table 5.1). Long-term sulfisoxazole is partly effective in preventing recurring attacks of acute otitis media (Liston *et al.* 1983). Adenoidectomy tends not to be helpful but has indication if secretory otitis media co-exists. The use of pneumococcal vaccine (Mäkelä *et al.* 1980) has no practical application at present.

Decongestant/Antihistamine	Effect
When developed a cold	Did not prevent acute otitis media
In the treatment of acute otitis media	No acute benefit
	Did not prevent subsequent acute otitis media
	Did not prevent subsequent secretory otitis media
In the treatment of secretory otitis media	No benefit
Mucolytics	
In the treatment of secretory otitis media	Some benefit

Table 5.1 Summary of the effects of oral decongestant/antihistamine mixtures, and mucolytics

CHRONIC OTITIS MEDIA

Chronic otitis media follows untreated or inappropriately treated acute otitis media. A continuing discharge causes fibrosis of the perforation margin and prevents natural closure. The patient exhibits recurring episodes of foul-smelling discharge which represent a flare-up of infection, and these episodes are interspersed with periods of quiescence which in adults may be prolonged.

Chronic otitis media is associated with a degree of deafness related to the extent of middle ear destruction, and may be complicated by cholesteatoma. Vertigo of recent onset indicates spread of infection to involve the vestibular labyrinth and requires urgent referral (Kerr 1984). Suppurative complications; lateral sinus thrombosis and brain abscess are possible, but rare.

Bacteriology

Pseudomonas aeruginosa, E. coli and *Proteus species* are common, and there may also be a mixed Gram-positive flora including *H. influenzae, Staph. aureus*, and β-haemolytic streptococci. The recorded incidence of anaerobic bacteria (Palva *et al.* 1969) is low.

Management and Antibiotic Use

Patients with chronic otitis media need referral, and long-term management is undertaken by the ENT department. The basis of treatment is periodic removal of debris by suction under microscopic view (aural toilet). Mastoidectomy is sometimes necessary, and in favourable circumstances tympanoplasty may be considered. Attention is given to adenoids, sinuses and tonsils if relevant.

Antibiotics active against aerobic bacteria are of limited value (Browning *et al.* 1983), but topical antibiotic plus steroid, e.g. gentamicin and hydrocortisone (Gentisone HC) or clioquinol and flumethasone (Locorten-vioform) used for two or three weeks, usually after aural toilet, can be of value. They are better not used in children owing to the risk of VIII nerve toxicity.

Metronidazole active against anaerobic bacteria *can* be helpful, and in practice a flare-up of infection is sometimes effectively managed by the combined use of metronidazole and cefaclor, followed (in adults) by a topical antibiotic–steroid combination. If *Pseudomonas aeruginosa* is isolated from the discharge, aural toilet is preferable to the systemic use of relevant antibiotics, e.g. gentamicin, colistin or polymyxin.

REFERENCES

Bain, D. J. G. (1983). Can the clinical course of acute otitis media be modified by systemic decongestant or antihistamine treatment? *Br. Med. J.*, **287**, 654–656

Bain, J., Murphy, E. and Ross, F. (1985). Acute otitis media: clinical course among children who received a short course of high dose antibiotic. *Br. Med. J.*, **291**, 1243–1246

Barritt, P. W. and Darbyshire, P. J. (1984). Deafness after otitis media in general practice. *J. R. Coll. Gen. Pract.*, **34**, 92–94

Bell, S. M. and Plowman, D. (1980). Mechanisms of ampicillin resistance in Haemophilus influenzae from respiratory tract. *Lancet*, **1**, 279–280

Branefors-Helander, P., Dahlberg, T. and Nylén, O. (1975). A clinical, bacteriological and serological study of children with frequent episodes of acute otitis media. *Acta Otolaryngol.*, **80**, 399–409

British National Formulary (1984). No. 8, p. 186. British Medical Association and The Pharmaceutical Society of Great Britain

Brook, I. (1979). Otitis media in children: a prospective study of aerobic and anaerobic bacteriology. *The Laryngoscope*, **89**, 992–997

Browning, G. G., Picozzi, G. L., Calder, I. T. and Sweeny, G. (1983). Controlled trial of medical treatment of active chronic otitis media. *Br. Med. J.*, **287**, 1024–1025

Grönroos, P. and Karma, P. (1980). Pneumococcal vaccine and otitis media. *Lancet*, **2**, 547–551

van Buchem, F. L., Dunk, J. H. M. and van't Hof, M. A. (1981). Therapy of acute otitis media: myringotomy, antibiotics, or neither? *Lancet*, **2**, 883–887

Cantekin, E. I., Mandel, E. M., Bluestone, C. D., Rockette, H. E., Paradise, J. L., Stool, S. E., Fria, T. J. and Rogers, K. D. (1983). Lack of efficacy of a decongestant-antihistamine combination for otitis media with effusion ("secretory" otitis media) in children. *N. Engl. J. Med.*, **308**, 297–301

Chaput de Saintonge, D. M., Levine, D. F., Temple Savage, I., Burgess, G. W. S., Sharp, J., Mayhew, S. R., Sadler, M. G., Moody, R., Griffiths, R., Griffiths, S. and Meadows, G. (1982). Trial of three-day and ten-day courses of amoxycillin in otitis media. *Br. Med. J.*, **284**, 1078–1081

Grace, A., Kalinkiewicz, M. and Drake-Lee, A. B. (1984). Covert manifestations of child abuse. *Br. Med. J.*, **289**, 1041–1042

Halsted, C., Lepow, M. L., Balassanian, N., Emmerich, J. and Wolinsky, E. (1968). Clinical observations, microbiology and evaluation of therapy. *Am. J. Dis. Child.*, **115**, 542–551

Howard, J. E., Nelson, J. D., Clahsen, J. and Hinton Jackson, L. (1976). Otitis media of infancy and early childhood. A double-blind study of four treatment regimens. *Am. J. Dis. Child.*, **130**, 965–970

Howie, V. M. and Ploussard, J. H. (1972). Efficacy of fixed combination antibiotics versus separate components in otitis media. *Clinical Pediatrics*, **11**, 205–214

Howie, V. M., Ploussard, J. H. and Lester, R. L. (1970). Otitis media: a clinical and bacteriological correlation. *Pediatrics*, **45**, 29–35

Ingvarsson, L. and Lundgren, K. (1982). Penicillin treatment of acute otitis media in children. A study of duration of treatment. *Acta Otolaryngol.*, **94**, 283–287

John, W. R. B. and Vallé-Jones, J. C. (1983). Treatment of otitis media in children. A comparison between cefaclor and amoxycillin. *The Practitioner*, **227**, 1805–1809

Kerr, A. I. G. (1984). Ear Infections. *The Physician*, **2**, 451–454

Klein, J. O. and Teele, D. W. (1976). Isolation of viruses and mycoplasmas from middle ear effusions. A review. *Ann. Otol. Rhinol. Laryngol.*, **85** (Suppl. 25), 140–144

Lim, D. J., Lewis, D. M., Schram, J. L. and Birck, H. G. (1980). Antibiotic-resistant bacteria in otitis media with effusion. *Acta Otol. Rhinol. Laryngol.*, **98** (Suppl. 68), 278–280

Liston, T. E., Foshee, W. S. and Pierson, W. D. (1983). Sulfisoxazole chemoprophylaxis for frequent otitis media. *Pediatrics*, **71**, 524–530

Mäkelä, P. H., Sibakov, M., Herva, E., Henrichsen, J., Luotonen, J., Timonen, M., Leinonen, M., Koskela, M., Pukander, J., Pöntynen, S., Meistrup-Larsen, K. I., Sorensen, H., Johnsen, N. J., Thomsen, J., Mygind, N. and Sederberg-Olsen, J. (1983). Two versus seven days penicillin treatment for acute otitis media. *Acta Otolaryngol.*, **96**, 99–104

Mygind, N., Meistrup-Larsen, K. I., Thomsen, J., Thomsen, V. F., Josefsson, K. and Sorensen, H. (1981). Penicillin in acute otitis media: a double-blind placebo-controlled trial. *Clin. Otolaryngol.*, **6**, 5–13

Olson, A. L., Klein, S. W., Charney, E., MacWhinney, J. B., McInery, T. K., Miller, R. L., Nazarian, L. F. and Cunningham, D. (1978). Prevention and therapy of serous otitis media by oral decongestant: a double blind study in pediatric practice. *Pediatrics*, **61**, 679–683

Palva, T., Karja, J., Palva, A. and Raunio, V. (1969). Bacteria in the chronic ear. *Pract. Oto-Rhino-Laryngol.*, **31**, 30–45

Philpott-Howard, J. and Williams, J. D. (1982). Increase in antibiotic resistance in *Haemophilus influenzae* in the United Kingdom since 1977: report of a study group. *Br. Med. J.*, **284**, 1597–1599

Poole, P. M. and Tobin, J. O'H. (1973). Viral and epidemiological findings in MRC/PHLS surveys of respiratory disease in hospital and general practice. *Postgrad. Med. J.*, **49**, 778–787

Randall, J. E. and Hendley, J. O. (1979). A decongestant–antihistamine mixture in the prevention of otitis media in children with colds. *Pediatrics*, **63**, 483–485

Rowe, D. S. (1975). Acute suppurative otitis media. *Pediatrics*, **56**, 285–294

Schwartz, R. H. and Rodriguez, W. J. (1981). Acute otitis media in children eight years old and older: a reappraisal of the role of *Haemophilus influenzae*. *Am. J. Otolaryngol.*, **2**, 19–21

Schwartz, R., Rodriguez, W. J., Khan, W. N. and Ross, S. (1977). Acute purulent otitis media in children older than 5 years. Incidence of Haemophilus as a causative organism. *J. Am. Med. Assoc.*, **238**, 1032–1033

Shurin, P. A., Pelton, S. I., Donner, A. and Klein, J. O. (1979). Persistence of middle-ear effusion after acute otitis media in children. *N. Engl. J. Med.*, **300**, 1121–1123

Taylor, P. H. and Dareshani, N. (1975). s-Carboxy-methyl-cysteine syrup in secretory otitis media. *Br. J. Clin. Pract.*, **29**, 177–180

6

Sinusitis

Clinical Features – Bacteriology – Management and Antibiotic Use

The diagnosis of sinusitis is not always easy because the sinuses cannot be looked at like the throat and ear, nor listened to like the chest. Difficulty can also arise in relating what is actually seen in general practice to what is written in books and journals. The general practitioner will often see adults with maxillary sinusitis (acute and chronic) but acute maxillary sinusitis in children is uncommon, and frontal sinusitis is rarely seen. Although it may seem wrong to say it, a general practitioner would seem able to practice medicine adequately without acknowledging the existence of ethmoid or sphenoidal sinusitis.

One explanation may be that chronic ethmoid sinusitis in adults is associated with nasal polyps, and it is these latter which are recognized by the general practitioner, while in children chronic ethmoid and/or maxillary sinusitis are overshadowed by the clinical features, for example, of adenoidal hyperplasia, and remain unrecognized unless the sinuses are X-rayed.

A further explanation may lie in the fact that pansinusitis is not uncommon, and that adequate treatment of maxillary sinusitis is the key to overall sinus management. In an extreme degree this means that in addition to drainage of another sinus, adequate ventilation and drainage of the maxillary sinus is necessary as well. In a milder form, it is possible that treatment ostensibly given for maxillary sinusitis will also control the other sinuses.

Age Incidence and Pneumatization

Both maxillary and ethmoid sinuses are present at birth and enlarge with growth. Pneumatization occurs early, and acute maxillary sinusitis can occur in children as young as 18 months (Wald *et al.* 1981). The sphenoidal sinus achieves clinical significance at the age of four or five years and the frontal sinus is pneumatized late, e.g. age 10–12 years. Frontal sinusitis therefore occurs in teenagers and adults.

Antecedent Causes

Sinusitis represents a secondary bacterial infection induced by inadequate drainage, and viral infections are the most common antecedent cause. Mechanical factors may alone underly sinusitis or allow a viral infection to more readily impair drainage.

Mechanical factors include septal deviation, nasal injury, nasal polyps, allergic rhinitis, vasomotor rhinitis, adenoidal hyperplasia, and foreign body. Sinusitis is not uncommon in patients with cystic fibrosis. Sinusitis of dental origin may be anaerobic in nature, and maxillary infection can be caused by an acute peri-apical abscess, a dentigerous cyst, a periodontal abscess, or by dental extraction.

CLINICAL FEATURES

The clinical features embrace antecedent causes, the general features of a collection of pus which cannot drain, the local features of whichever sinus is involved and rarely complicating features.

Acute Sinusitis

Maxillary

Following a cold or influenza or 'flu-like illness, a typical story is for the 'cold-in-the-nose' component of the illness to persist, and for the features of sinusitis to develop about ten days after the start of the illness. This is in contrast to the often earlier recognition of complicating pneumonia in a 'flu-like illness. The patient with acute maxillary sinusitis is usually less ill than the patient with pneumonia, and a high temperature is uncommon. Another illness pattern sometimes seen in a respiratory viral infection is recrudescence of pyrexia after initial subsidence, and this later pyrexia also reflects a secondary bacterial infection which could be either pneumonia or sinusitis.

Pain overlying the sinus is made worse by bending down; the upper teeth may ache, and percussion of these teeth and of the antrum itself can cause pain. The nose is likely to be blocked on the affected side with a degree of nasal discharge dependent upon the extent of drainage. The involved inferior turbinate is congested, and if a view can be obtained, pus may be visible in the middle meatus. The severity of pain and illness is dependent upon the extent of drainage, and the clinical picture commonly seen is more subacute than acute. Acute maxillary sinusitis is uncommon in children and may be associated with ipsilateral conjunctivitis, and may present as PUO.

Frontal

Acute frontal sinusitis causes generalized headache with pain over the forehead and the patient is likely to be pyrexial and ill. The upper eyelid on the affected side may become red and oedematous and oedema may be present over the eyebrow. The medial aspect of the supraorbital rim is tender. The pain sometimes decreases by mid-day, because drainage is more effective when upright. Infection in the corresponding maxillary sinus is usually present as well. Acute frontal sinusitis may present as a complication.

Ethmoidal and Sphenoidal

Acute ethmoidal infection is likely to be recognized only when pus reaches the orbit causing a periosteal abscess with orbital symptoms and signs, but acute ethmoid sinusitis can occur in association with acute maxillary sinusitis. Acute sphenoidal sinusitis occurs as part of a more generalized sinusitis, and the pain is felt in the centre skull, and referred to the temple, back of neck, sides of neck and behind the ears (Hall and Coleman 1975).

Suppurative Complications

When rarely occurring, these complications are reflected in the clinical presentation of sinusitis, and include orbital cellulitis or abscess, frontal extradural abscess, meningitis, brain abscess of the frontal lobe, cavernous sinus thrombosis and osteomyelitis of the frontal bone (Pott's puffy tumour). Cerebral abscess of sinus origin is likely to have an anaerobic bacterial component (Grace and Drake-Lee 1984), and deteriorating vision with orbital infection demands urgent sinus drainage if blindness is to be prevented (Smelt and Migdal 1983).

Chronic Sinusitis

Adults with chronic sinusitis are likely to have a story of recurring episodes of acute sinusitis and evidence of an antecedent cause as already outlined. Diagnosis is by X-ray. In between acute episodes, the symptoms may suggest a cold which does not clear up. Children usually over the age of three years can have chronic sinusitis in association with adenoidal hyperplasia, recurrent otitis media, glue-ear and allergic rhinitis, but it is problematical how often it in fact occurs. The clinical picture reflects the underlying cause, and is usually manifest by nasal obstruction and a persistent 'cold' with perhaps cough. X-ray is necessary for diagnosis.

BACTERIOLOGY

Fungal sinusitis can rarely occur (Wright 1981), but for practical purposes both acute and chronic sinusitis reflect secondary bacterial infection. Bacteriological data is obtained by antral wash or direct antral swab, but aspiration of the middle meatus (Bridger 1980) furnishes a method of equal reliability.

Acute Sinusitis

A wide range of aerobic bacteria are found in acute sinusitis, and isolations are often multiple, but *Str. pneumoniae* and *H. influenzae* predominate. Children differ little from adults, with the exception that *Str. pneumoniae* and *H. influenzae* together comprise two thirds of the bacterial isolations, representing a slightly higher incidence than occurring in adults. The incidence of anaerobioc bacteria in acute sinusitis is low.

Staphylococcus aureus

The incidence was low in adults assessed by needle puncture of the antrum (Evans *et al.* 1975) and absent in children undergoing sinus aspiration (Wald *et al.* 1981), but Lystad *et al.* (1961) found *Staph. aureus* to be the most commonly isolated organism after *H. influenzae* and *Str. pneumoniae*, and an even higher incidence was recorded by Bridger (1980) whose findings suggested pathogenicity. This implication of a highish incidence of *Staph. aureus* means that the bacteriology of acute sinusitis is different from that occurring in throat, ear or chest, and may therefore reflect a different antibiotic emphasis in treatment.

Chronic Sinusitis

The particular feature of chronic sinusitis is the high incidence of anaerobic bacteria in both adults (Frederick and Braude 1974) and children (Brook 1981), and these findings again have relevance to antibiotic emphasis. Aerobic bacteria include α-haemolytic streptococci, *Staph. aureus* and *H. influenzae*.

MANAGEMENT AND ANTIBIOTIC USE

Acute Sinusitis

Illness Management

Treatment entails the use of an antibiotic and a nasal decongestant, e.g. ephedrine nasal drops. A majority of the patients (adults and children) will respond to this combination but hospital admission is advisable for the rarely occurring acute frontal sinusitis.

The management of acute sinusitis is governed by two principles. Firstly, if there is no reasonably prompt response to treatment or if acute sinusitis seems to be recurring, then referral for antral washouts at an early stage will prevent chronic sinusitis and the possible need for difficult definitive surgery (Coleman 1975). Secondly, the antrum is the key to all the sinuses, and adequate antral drainage is necessary irrespective of treatment to other sinuses.

Antibiotic Use

There is no issue about antibiotic need, and the only question relates to choice. Doxycycline is more effective than other antibiotics. Agbim (1974) compared the use of seven days' doxycycline with seven days' ampicillin in 44 adults aged 16–55 years with acute sinusitis, and demonstrated a good or very good response in only 35% of those treated with ampicillin, whereas 90% responded in the doxycycline-treated group. This effect is borne out in clinical practice. Anecdotally, patients failing to respond to a conventional antibiotic will then respond rapidly to doxycycline, and if a patient has once had doxycycline for an attack of acute sinusitis, will ask specifically for it should a further attack occur. Patients can also *develop* acute sinusitis while on a different antibiotic.

The particular value of doxycycline is something of a paradox. Theoretically, the ideal antibiotic should be active against *Str. pneumoniae* and *H. influenzae and Staph. aureus*. Either cefaclor or co-trimoxazole would seem to be ideal choices. The poor results with ampicillin (Agbim 1974) are no surprise because ampicillin has little activity against *Staphylococcus aureus*. The same poor result would be expected with amoxycillin, but theoretically augmentin (clavulanate-potentiated amoxycillin) should be much more effective. Erythromycin is not an ideal choice, despite its activity against *Staph. aureus*, owing to its reduced activity against *H. influenzae*.

Doxycycline does have activity against all three bacteria, but sensitivity is not complete. It is possible, however, that the particular value of doxycycline is related less to bacterial sensitivities, and is more dependent upon its particular ability to penetrate purulent secretions. It would be for this same reason that doxycycline can be of value in bronchiectasis (Chapter 11).

Doxycycline is also effective in children, and acute sinusitis in children represents one of the two situations in clinical practice when it is justifiable to use a tetracycline despite the risk of staining the secondary dentition. (The other situation is an atypical pneumonia.) If the use of doxycycline is considered inadvisable (e.g. pregnancy) an alternative choice may be made from cefaclor, co-trimoxazole or augmentin.

Chronic Sinusitis

If four or five antral washouts fail to produce a completely clear lavage, definitive surgery may be undertaken. Chronic sinusitis requires management by the ENT department, but an acute flare-up of infection might well be managed at home. Owing to the known high incidence of anaerobic bacteria in chronic sinusitis, the additional use of metronidazole could be beneficial.

REFERENCES

Agbim, O. G. (1974). A comparative trial of doxycycline ("Vibramycin") and ampicillin in the treatment of acute sinusitis. *Curr. Med. Res. Opinion*, **2**, 291–294

Bridger, R. C. (1980). Sinusitis: an improved régime of investigation for the clinical laboratory. *J. Clin. Path.*, **33**, 276–281

Brook, I. (1981). Bacteriologic features of chronic sinusitis in children. *J. Am. Med. Assoc.*, **246**, 967–969

Coleman, B. H. (1975). Sinusitis. *The Practitioner*, **215**, 725–731

Evans, F. O. Jr., Syndor, J. B., Moore, W. E. C., Moore, G. R., Manwaring, J. L., Brill, A. H., Jackson, R. T., Hanna, S., Skaar, J. S., Holdeman, L. V., Fitz-Hugh, G. S., Sande, M. A. and Gwaltney, J. M. Jr. (1975). Sinusitis of the maxillary antrum. *N. Engl. J. Med.*, **293**, 735–739

Frederick, J. and Braude, A. I. (1974). Anaerobic infection of the paranasal sinuses. *N. Engl. J. Med.*, **290**, 135–137

Grace, A. and Drake-Lee, A. (1984). Role of anaerobes in cerebral abscesses of sinus origin. *Br. Med. J.*, **288**, 758–759

Hall, I. S. and Coleman, B. H. (1975). *Diseases of the Nose, Throat and Ear.* p. 63. (Edinburgh, London and New York: Churchill Livingstone)

Lystad, A., Berdal, P. and Lund-Iversen, L. (1961). The bacterial flora of sinusitis with an in-vitro study of the bacterial resistance to antibiotics. *Acta Oto-laryngol.*, **188** (Suppl.) 390–399

Smelt, G. J. C. and Migdal, C. S. (1983). Acute blinding sinusitis. *Br. Med. J.*, **287**, 1051–1052

Wald, E. R., Milmoe, G. J., Bowen, A'D., Ledesma-Medina, J., Salamon, N. and Bluestone, C. D. (1981). Acute maxillary sinusitis in children. *N. Engl. J. Med.*, **304**, 749–754

Wright, D. (1981). Sinusitis acute and chronic. *The Practitioner*, **225**, 1555–1564

7
Laryngitis

Croup – Hoarseness or Loss of Voice

Acute laryngitis is nearly always caused by a viral infection, and in small children is manifest as croup, whereas adults exhibit hoarseness or loss of voice. This age distinction is not absolute; children will sometimes have a hoarse voice, and croup can rarely occur in older children and adults.

CROUP

Croup is a colloquial term for inspiratory stridor, and for practical purposes represents either acute viral laryngo-tracheitis or acute epiglottitis.

Acute Viral Laryngo-tracheitis

This is by far the commonest cause and represents the croup which is seen several times each winter in general practice among small children aged usually between one and three years. Pathologically the inflammation is *below* the vocal cords (Morus Jones 1975). Parainfluenza viruses are most often the cause, but the whole range of common viruses can be responsible (Poole and Tobin 1973) including measles.

Acute Epiglottitis

This is a rare cause but will always be in the back of one's mind when managing croup. Acute epiglottitis is a bacterial infection caused by *Haemophilus influenzae* type B, and pathologically there is oedema and inflammation *above* the vocal cords (Morus Jones 1975) affecting the epiglottis and laryngeal inlet. Any minor change can result in total blockage, and it is for this reason, despite its rarity as a cause of croup, that inspection of the throat with a tongue depressor should *not* be undertaken in small children with croup.

Clinical Features

Typically the child goes to bed at the usual time and then wakes later in the evening (e.g. 11.00 pm or midnight) with croup. Clinical examination is invariably negative but the throat is not looked at; quite apart from the risk of using a tongue depressor in the rarely occurring acute epiglottitis, attempts to view the throat in a small child will cause distress which is the exact opposite of the aims of management. The child should be examined with a minimum of fuss.

Almost all instances will recover promptly in a warm, moist atmosphere. Failure to do so will indicate the possibility of acute epiglottitis or a severe degree of laryngo-tracheitis which can itself rarely require intubation also. There is no early reliable guide to indicate whether intubation might become necessary. Initial severity of the croup does not distinguish acute laryngo-tracheitis from acute epiglottitis (Couriel 1984), and the presence or absence of a prodromal respiratory illness is also no guide (Welch and Price 1983).

Impending laryngeal obstruction causes hypoxaemia resulting in restlessness, anxiety, increasing tachycardia and tachypnoea. Associated retraction of the chest wall includes intercostal recession, sternal recession and supra-sternal recession. Cyanosis is a late feature. The child with acute epiglottitis typically sits and leans forwards with an extended neck, drools saliva, and is pale, ill, and pyrexial. The child should *not* be laid down because this might cause total airway obstruction. A high temperature is unusual in acute laryngo-tracheitis, and is suggestive of acute epiglottitis.

Acute epiglottitis in adults causes a sudden onset of throat pain with increasingly painful dysphagia. Stridor is a late finding (McDonald 1984).

Management and Antibiotic Use

In addition to specific therapeutic measures, management entails an awareness of the rare need for intubation. Immediate hospital admission is advisable if there is no improvement after one hour in a steamy atmosphere.

Steam

It may be possible to make the diagnosis from the story given over the telephone, and advice may then be given *over the 'phone* to sit with the child in the bathroom with the hot bath tap turned on because this is the most effective way of placing the child swiftly in a warm, steamy environment. In this manner, the child will already be improved by the time the doctor arrives at the house.

An alternative method of steam utilization is to boil a kettle in whichever room the child happens to be in. This method gives a steamy environment of less density but is adequate alone in the absence of piped hot water and may follow the brief sojourn in the bathroom when piped hot water *is* available. There is no requirement for the kettle to be near the child or near the bed in the bedroom; the object is to steam the atmosphere of the room. The kettle is placed in the corner of the room on the floor, well away from the child in order to avoid burning by accident, and is allowed to boil and puff out steam for three or four minutes. This short duration is perfectly adequate. The parent sits by the kettle during the entire three or four minutes, again in order to avoid accidents. The kettle is then removed from the room.

The view that use of an electric kettle is impracticable and unsafe (Bacon 1978) is entirely without foundation. The kettle is not left on all night; the parents do not lose sleep by persistently refillng the kettle during the night, and the furniture does not rot. Henry (1983) agrees that a warm, moist atmosphere helps, but questions whether the warmth and moisture is the operative factor, or whether the associated comfort and reassurance is more important. If the parents are reassured and freed from fear the child will certainly settle more quickly, and the child also gains comfort from sitting with his mother.

Sedation

Sedation is not essential, but a single dose of phenergan or dichloralphenazone (Welldorm) from the doctor's bag helps.

Antibiotic Use

The rarely occurring acute epiglottitis needs an antibiotic effective against *H. influenzae* type B. This organism has a resistance rate of 14.0% to ampicillin (and amoxycillin) which is higher than the overall resistance rate of 6.6% among other strains of *H. influenzae* (Philpott-Howard and Williams 1982), and in hospital the immediate use of chloramphenicol is appropriate (Mier and Shanson 1984).

In the general practice setting, the question is whether a child with croup should be given an antibiotic, recognizing that almost all will reflect acute laryngo-tracheitis, and that the chest will invariably be clear. Acute laryngo-tracheitis is a viral infection and the extent to which secondary bacterial invasion of the larynx might occur is uncertain because laryngeal swabs are never undertaken in the less severe illness. It is of relevance that children with severe acute laryngo-tracheitis needing intubation (Welch and Price 1983) were managed without antibiotics and suffered no detriment.

In conclusion, the child with croup caused by acute laryngo-tracheitis probably gains little benefit from antibiotic use, but antibiotics tend to be prescribed because the situation causes fear and because there is a very small risk of acute epiglottitis. While such prescribing has little scientific justification, it cannot be too harshly criticized. The drug chosen should be effective against *H. influenzae*; either cefaclor or co-trimoxazole would be more appropriate than ampicillin or amoxycillin owing to the incidence of resistant strains.

An Emergency Airway

The need is exceptionally rare, but a large-bore needle, e.g. Medicut size 14, should be carried in the doctor's bag. The needle is inserted through the crico-thyroid membrane.

Alternatively, a laryngotomy may be made, again through the crico-thyroid membrane. A cushion is placed under the shoulders and the neck kept extended and the skin taut. After a vertical incision through the skin, the crico-thyroid membrane may be entered by a direct thrust. The knife is then rotated through 90° in order to open up the space. The airway can be maintained by a convenient tube, e.g. drinking straw or barrel of a ball-point pen. To minimize bleeding into the trachea the patient should then be placed on his side and with a 30° head-down tilt, and maintained in this position until arriving at hospital (Howells

1984). A Portex Minitracheotomy Kit, for example, obviates the need to use a household knife and to find a convenient tube.

Steroids

The role of steroids in acute epiglottitis and severe laryngo-tracheitis is controversial. The intention is to reduce laryngeal oedema, but in 50 children with acute epiglottitis (33) and acute laryngo-tracheitis (17) needing intubation, Welch and Price (1983) found no benefit. It is therefore inadvisable for a general practitioner to give an injection of hydrocortisone before transfer to hospital, because the resulting distress to the child could outweigh its benefit.

Other Causes and Differential Diagnosis

Pseudomembranous Croup

Pseudomembranous croup is a severe form of laryngo-tracheo-bronchitis tending to occur in older children and exhibiting a longer prodromal phase. The obstruction is subglottic and *Staphylococcus aureus* is the most commonly identified bacterium. 'Bacterial tracheitis' (Sofer *et al.* 1983) is likely to be the same disorder.

Supraglottic Foreign Body

The patient, previously well, suddenly develops noisy ineffectual respiratory efforts, and becomes cyanosed. The Heimlich manoeuvre may be used, and theoretically if this fails, an emergency airway through the crico-thyroid membrane is necessary, but time available is minimal.

Congenital Laryngeal Stridor

The stridor develops shortly after birth and persists for several months, with eventual disappearance at the age of 18 months to two years (Barnes and Roberton 1979). The cause is laryngomalacia resulting in collapse of the soft supra-laryngeal and laryngeal tissue during inspiration. Feeding may be associated with cyanotic attacks, and upper respiratory illness may exacerbate the stridor.

Tetany

Intermittent stridor may rarely be caused by tetany (Goodall 1973) and is most likely to occur in dark-skinned immigrant babies in whom Vitamin D absorption from the skin is low.

Asthma

Parents will sometimes think that their child has asthma when croup occurs. A careful history and a little time spent with the child will clarify whether or not the noise being made is the very characteristic sound of croup.

HOARSENESS OR LOSS OF VOICE

Acute Laryngitis

Acute laryngitis in adults and older children is caused by the same wide range of viruses and results in hoarseness or loss of voice of short duration, e.g. a few days. These age groups exhibit a further difference from the croup of small children in that the causative virus is more in evidence. Patients will have, for example, a cold, cough, sore throat, perhaps pyrexia, or a full 'flu-like illness or influenza. An associated tracheitis results in retrosternal pain. Other causes of acute laryngitis include sudden exposure, tobacco, and overuse of the voice, but occur much less often.

Management and Antibiotic Use

Steam

The need for steam is less pressing in adults and older children but can bring relief. The most convenient method is to pour boiling water into a bowl or saucepan, and to inhale the warm moisture which emanates from its surface.

Antibiotic Use

The same dilemma applies as already discussed in relation to antibiotic use in croup. The cause is viral and there is no certainty that secondary bacterial infection occurs. There is probably no scientific justification for antibiotic use but a husky or lost voice is an emotive prescribing situation. The association of a painful tracheitis perhaps lends greater justification to prescription. If an antibiotic is given, the choice should again have activity against *Haemophilus influenzae*.

Persistent Hoarseness

If hoarseness persists for six weeks, the patient must be quickly referred in order to determine the presence or absence of other causes, in particular laryngeal tumour.

REFERENCES

Bacon, L. (1978). Treatment of minor respiratory illness in group practice. *J. R. Coll. Gen. Pract.*, **28**, 758

Barnes, N.D. and Roberton, N.R.C. (1979). Upper respiratory tract infections. *Update*, **18**, 1131–1140

Couriel, J. (1984). Acute stridor in the pre-school child. *Br. Med. J.*, **288**, 1162

Goodall, J. (1973). Persistent or recurrent cough in children: causes and management. *Update*, **7**, 1539–1550

Henry, R. (1983). Moist air in the treatment of laryngo-tracheitis. *Arch. Dis. Child.*, **58**, 577

Howells, T.H. (1984). Disaster at the dining table. *Br. Med. J.*, **289**, 511–512

McDonald, K. (1984). Acute epiglottitis in adults. *N. Z. Med. J.*, **97**, 701

Mier, A. and Shanson, D.C. (1984). Ampicillin-resistant *Haemophilus influenzae* epiglottis and pericarditis in an adult. *Lancet*, **11**, 817

Morus Jones, H. (1975). Acute epiglottitis. *The Practitioner*, **215**, 732–739

Philpott-Howard, J. and Williams, J.D. (1982). Increase in antibiotic resistant *Haemophilus influenzae* in the United Kingdom since 1977: a report of a study group. *Br. Med. J.*, **284**, 1597–1599

Poole, P.M. and Tobin, J. O'H. (1973). Viral and epidemiological findings in MRC/PHLS surveys of respiratory disease in hospital and general practice. *Postgrad. Med. J.*, **49**, 778–787

Sofer, S., Duncan, P. and Chernick, V. (1983). Bacterial tracheitis – an old disease rediscovered. *Clin. Pediatr.*, **22**, 407–411

Welch, D.B. and Price, D.G. (1983). Acute epiglottitis and severe croup. Experience in two English regions. *Anaesthesia*, **38**, 754–759

8
Coughs and Colds

The Acute Cough - Cold in the Nose - Persistent Cough in Children - Persistent Cough in Adults - The Absent Cough

Treatment is dependent upon cause.

Assessment of the Patient

As always, a history is taken and the patient examined. In children, the five features to enquire about are cold and cough, vomiting and diarrhoea, and pyrexia. Dependent upon age, other symptoms may be presented or should be enquired about, namely earache, sore throat, headache and abdominal pain. The chronological order of symptom development should be recorded and symptom severity noted. Clinical examination should embrace ears, throat, cervical nodes, chest and sometimes the abdomen, but in toddlers and infants it may not always be necessary to look at the throat (Chapter 4). Examination of the chest automatically allows visualization of any rash. If a 'flu illness seems likely, additional enquiry is necessary relating to foreign travel, occupation, and animal or bird contact (Chapter 14).

This assessment will clarify the duration of both cold and cough, establish the presence or absence of associated illness features, and identify any abnormal physical signs.

THE ACUTE COUGH

Common Viral Causes

These illnesses are by far the commonest cause of cough, and it is exceptional for the cough to occur alone. A cold in the nose is invariably associated and other illness features are usually present as well. There is ample evidence (Wilks 1973, Poole and Tobin 1973, Higgins 1974) that a wide range of viruses may be responsible in both adults and children, including Influenza A, Influenza B, rhinoviruses, adenoviruses, enteroviruses, respiratory syncytial virus (RSV), parainfluenza viruses and herpes simplex. The influenza viruses and RSV appear in the winter and early spring, enteroviruses mainly during the summer and autumn, and rhinoviruses, adenoviruses and herpes simplex at any time of the year. Parainfluenza viruses also appear at any time of the year but outbreaks tend to have summer peaks and tend not to coincide with RSV (Martin *et al.* 1978).

There is wide variation in the complexity of illness because each virus is capable of a wide illness spectrum. In adults, for example, Influenza A can cause anything from a mild cold and cough to a full influenzal illness. The variation in the complexity of illness is also dependent upon age. Small children are limited in the extent to which they can complain of symptoms, and in the toddler the usual illness is a simple cold and cough, but there will sometimes also be pyrexia, non-specific vomiting and diarrhoea. Otitis media is a common complication. In slightly older children, e.g. aged 3–6 years, sore throat, headache and non-specific abdominal pain may be additional symptoms and tonsillitis will sometimes be seen. Sinusitis occasionally occurs, and a chest infection may be present at any age.

When pyrexia occurs in 'simple respiratory illness' (cold, cough etc. without 'flu and without chest infection) it is possible to define two different illness patterns. These are the same patterns which are seen in the 'flu-like illness, and the similarity is no surprise because the 'flu-like illness is simply a more severe and complex version of the same viral cause. In one pattern the pyrexia may be present from the start of the illness, and in the other pattern the pyrexia develops up to a few days after illness onset, being preceded, for example, by cold and cough. These two different patterns seem unrelated to any particular viral cause, but do have relevance to antibiotic use.

The cough itself also has two patterns, being sometimes present from the start of the illness but quite commonly having a delayed onset.

These patterns also seem unrelated to any particular viral cause, but again, have relevance to antibiotic use.

Children with cough will often vomit. This is commonly non-specific but also represents the child's method of getting rid of the sputum. Diarrhoea is occasionally seen, particularly in adenovirus or enterovirus infections.

Antibiotic Use

With reference to the cough itself, the decision for or against antibiotic use has to depend upon the presence or absence of abnormal signs in the chest. This rule of thumb approach makes sense because trying to relate pathological terms to clinical findings can be difficult, but there are two exceptions. Pneumonia which does need an antibiotic can occasionally present without abnormality on auscultation, and in the reverse situation, the 'chest full of signs' occurring in wheezy bronchitis might be managed without antibiotics.

In the management of respiratory viral infections, two situations commonly occur and may be seen in any age group. An example is the child who has had a cold and cough for two or three days, and then develops pyrexia (delayed pyrexia pattern). The advent of pyrexia is usually the event which brings the child to the doctor, and the pyrexia *could* represent otitis media or a chest infection, but often no cause is found. In this event the parents can be reassured that the pyrexia represents the normal course of the illness and unnecessary antibiotic withheld. Depending upon clinical judgement, the child would probably be followed-up.

The other situation is the patient who has had a cold and perhaps pyrexia for one or two days, and then develops a cough and presents for this reason. The adult may comment that 'it has gone down onto my chest', and indeed it may have, but often, and particularly in children and younger adults, clinical examination will be negative and the delayed advent of cough represents the normal illness pattern. Again, unnecessary antibiotic use can be avoided, and both situations emphasize the value to be gained from recognizing patterns of illness.

Over and above these guidelines, an antibiotic may sometimes be felt to be justifiable despite a clear chest, if the cough is particularly 'bad' or 'chesty' or 'croupy'.

Purulent sputum in adults is an emotive indication for antibiotic use. Chest infections resulting in purulent sputum do of course justify antibiotic use, but purulent sputum is not an indication in an otherwise healthy person with an acute viral illness and a clear chest (Stott and West 1976).

Antibiotic Choice

If the patient has a frank chest infection, antibiotic choice follows the guidelines for pneumonia (Chapter 10). If the chest is clear, a broad spectrum antibiotic will usually be chosen, e.g. ampicillin, amoxycillin or co-trimoxazole. If the reason for antibiotic use is to abort pertussis (see later) then erythromycin would usually be chosen.

Cough Medicines and Sedatives

In the acute cough which may last up to about two weeks, the value of cough medicines at any age is very limited. If a patient or parent wishes to use a cough medicine, then they may do so but should purchase it. If an antibiotic *is* prescribed, the patient can be advised that their cough medicine will not 'fight' with the antibiotic. In infants and small toddlers it is wiser to avoid cough medicines altogether, and if a night sedative seems indicated, to use phenergan.

It is evident that if antibiotics are withheld and if cough medicines are viewed with scepticism, then there is little else to offer. This is the reality, and as discussed in Chapter 2, the doctor should not be afraid to state that there is no specific treatment and that the illness has to run its course. There is, however, one other management method which can help, namely steam.

Steam

Steam is best known for its use in croup, but can often be of great value for the acute cough which may be troublesome at night. The most convenient method for children is to steam the bedroom for 3–4 minutes before the child goes to bed, and then again for a further 3–4 minutes before the parents retire, using an electric kettle as detailed in Chapter 7. Adults may prefer to inhale moisture from the surface of a bowl of hot water.

Early Symptom of Another Cause
Measles

The initial cold, cough, pyrexia and perhaps conjunctivitis is indistinguishable from any other acute respiratory viral illness. Koplik's spots are seldom seen, and the diagnosis becomes suspect if the temperature persists to a third day without explanation, and then becomes evident when the rash appears on the fourth day.

Antibiotic Use

Neither pneumonia nor otitis media is prevented by early antibiotic use, and suspect measles should therefore be managed on a selective antibiotic basis like any other acute respiratory illness. An antibiotic might be given early before diagnosis, for the occasional tonsillitis occurring during the prodromal phase, or for an early complicating otitis media. If an antibiotic *is* used during the prodromal 'upper respiratory illness' phase of what is thought might represent early measles, then use of an antibiotic other than penicillin would help to reduce the possibility of confusion between exanthem and allergy, should a rash subsequently develop. In diagnosed measles, the child should be seen daily for two or three days, and a watch kept on ears and chest.

Rotavirus

The rotavirus is a common cause of gastro-enteritis particularly in children under the age of two years, but the diarrhoea and vomiting are commonly preceded by respiratory features, e.g. cold, cough, pyrexia and perhaps otitis media (Lewis *et al.* 1979).

Antibiotic Use

The initial respiratory illness is indistinguishable from any other acute respiratory viral illness and is managed in the same selective way.

Pertussis

The initial respiratory illness is indistinguishable from any other acute cough, is indistinguishable from any other acute respiratory viral illness, but the disease will be suspect if a pertussis outbreak is present in the community at the time.

Antibiotic Use

Trollfors and Rabo (1981) have demonstrated that erythromycin given within four days of onset of the catarrhal symptoms aborts the illness, and although these results were obtained in adults with whooping cough, it would seem reasonable to expect the disease in children to behave in the same way. This means that erythromycin has to be given at the cold/cough stage before the diagnosis is evident, and it may reasonably be given to all non-immunized children who present with a cold and cough during a pertussis outbreak.

Erythromycin may also be considered for adults presenting with cold and cough during a pertussis outbreak, because neither previous whooping cough nor immunization as a child will necessarily prevent re-infection in adults (Trollfors and Rabo 1981). The other uses of antibiotics in pertussis (prophylaxis, reducing infectivity and treating complications) are discussed subsequently.

Bronchitis, Bronchioliotis, Bronchiectasis and Pneumonia

These illnesses are discussed in the relevant chapters.

Mycoplasma Pneumoniae

Mycoplasma pneumoniae is known to cause an appreciable incidence of pneumonia in children, and it has been suggested that this organism could also be a common cause of simple respiratory illness. A study of relevant literature (Noah 1974, Krech *et al.* 1976, Mardh *et al.* 1976, Foy *et al.* 1979, Horn *et al.* 1979, Epidemiology 1980) suggests that *M. pneumoniae* is likely to cause an incidence of minor respiratory illness *during epidemics* and *among children*, but is less likely to be a significant cause in adults or in between epidemics. There would seem to be no justification for antibiotic use in children with simple respiratory illness on the grounds that a proportion are caused by

Mycoplasma pneumoniae, and the suggestion by McSherry (1981) that 'heavy colds' might justify antibiotic use for this reason is unsubstantiated.

Rare Causes

Inhaled Foreign Body

Children between six months and three years are most commonly affected (Moazam *et al.* 1983) and present with choking, subsequent cough and wheeze, and possibly cyanosis. The cough may however be delayed until a chest infection supervenes, or the child may present with a persistent cough. It is significant that the cough occurs without a cold, which is unusual in small children. Sometimes a wheeze is the only symptom. On examination a localized wheeze and reduced breath sounds will sometimes be heard, and X-ray may aid diagnosis.

Foreign Body in Ear or Nose

A reflex cough may be caused by a foreign body pushed hard up the nose or into the ear.

Cardiac Failure

Cardiac failure in children usually becomes manifest in infants under the age of six months who are then thought to have pneumonia. In adults, left ventricular failure may cause a cough.

Ascaris Lumbricoides

The larvae may cause transient respiratory symptoms while passing through the lungs.

COLD IN THE NOSE

The term cold will be used to mean cold in the nose.

Causes and Clinical Features

The causes are the same as the infective causes of the acute cough, as already outlined, and reflect the same clinical illnesses. Cold and cough nearly always occur together. In children under the age of four years, a cold will sometimes result in a profuse purulent nasal discharge from which *Streptococcus pneumoniae* and/or *Haemophilus influenzae* can be isolated, but it is uncertain whether these bacteria should be regarded as pathogenic.

Complications

Because a cold often forms part of a more complex illness, the patient needs a full assessment. In particular the cold itself can result in otitis media, conjunctivitis or sinusitis. Infants and small children do sometimes have a cold in the nose without any other illness feature, but this phenomenon in other age groups suggests a different diagnosis.

Differential Diagnosis

Adenoidal Hyperplasia

Children aged 2-7 years are affected most commonly and the particular features to look for are nasal obstruction, deafness, recurring otitis media and a persistent nasal discharge. The child mouth-breathes and snores at night but not all mouth-breathers have enlarged adenoids, and the nasal obstruction may not become evident until a viral infection causes additional inflammatory swelling of the adenoids resulting in a total nose block. A child who prefers to nose-breathe may then have major breathing problems at night.

Allergic Rhinitis

Allergic rhinitis is unlikely to be confused with a cold. There is no acute illness and nasal symptoms occur either seasonally (hay fever) or all the year round (perennial rhinitis). Both adults and children are affected, but allergic rhinitis does not commonly become evident until the child is three or four years of age, and adults will often 'grow out' of the disorder by middle age.

Sinusitis

A persistent nasal discharge may be caused by chronic sinusitis. An adult would probably have an associated nasal obstruction, e.g. polyp, septal deviation (Chapter 6) and a child adenoidal hyperplasia. Acute sinusitis can complicate a viral infection, e.g. cold, cough, 'flu-illness, and the 'cold in the nose' component of the illness then persists.

Vasomotor Rhinitis

Vasomotor rhinitis is uncommon and occurs in adults. It represents an imbalance of autonomic vascular innervation with an increased sensitivity to other stimuli, e.g. tobacco, alcohol, drugs, climate and hormonal disturbance.

Foreign Body and Tumour

A unilateral sero-sanguinous discharge in a child is likely to mean a foreign body, and in an adult may indicate a tumour.

Syphilis

Neonatal syphilis can present as snuffles and is more likely to be seen in developing countries or where antenatal care is inadequate.

Management and Antibiotic Use

Antibiotic Use

Cold in the nose when viewed as an individual illness feature, whether occurring along or as part of a more complex illness, does not justify antibiotic use except possibly in the small child with a purulent nasal discharge from which *Str. pneumoniae* and/or *H. influenzae* is isolated. The role of erythromycin in aborting pertussis has already been discussed, and it has already been argued that antibiotic use for colds on the grounds that some are caused by *Mycoplasma pneumoniae*, is unjustified.

Antiviral Drugs

Intra-nasal enviroxime has potential as an antirhinovirus agent (Phillpotts et al. 1981) and intra-nasal interferon shortens the duration of colds (Herzog et al. 1983). Neither agent has general clinical application at present and a problem with a virus-specific antiviral agent is the multiviral cause of colds.

Infants

The nose block caused by a cold causes greater problems in infants than in any other age group. Infants and very small children breathe almost exclusively through the nose, and its block interferes with both sleep and feeding. Interference with sleep results in a restless night for the child and a sleepless night for the parents. Interference with feeding could allow a degree of dehydration, and if the infant is being fed on unmodified milk formulae with a high sodium content (unlikely now), the dehydration could lead to hypernatraemia with a risk of brain damage or cot death.

Ephedrine nose drops are of considerable value and because the problem commonly arises during the evening, it is advisable for the doctor to carry a bottle in his bag. Excessive use of ephedrine nose drops can cause a shock-like state in infants and toddlers, and it is necessary to advise the parents when and how to instil them. The drops may be instilled into each nostril up to four times in the 24 hour period and should not exceed two drops each time. The parent is instructed to draw the fluid into the dropper and to then let most of the fluid fall back into the bottle so that a very small amount representing one or two drops remains in the bottom of the dropper. With the child lying prone and someone holding the head, the dropper is placed at the nostril entrance and the tiny amount squeezed in. The dropper is then loaded again for the other side. In this manner it is impossible to instil too much, and the right amount is put into the right place. The drops are usually instilled before the child is settled for the night, and the other instillations are generally made prior to some of the feeds.

Cot Death

Respiratory features are one of the factors contributing to the risk of cot death (Carpenter et al. 1979), caused in particular by respiratory syncytial and para-influenza viruses (Downham *et al*. 1975, Williams *et al*. 1984). Additionally, infants dying from hyperpyrexia induced by excessive clothing or an unduly warm environment commonly had an associated viral or bacterial infection (Stanton 1984).

Colds may seem to be trivial but a visit request (commonly in the evening) for an infant or very small child should be honoured because the advice and management given might be preventative. In addition to nose drops and advice about adequate hydration, the mother is advised to have the baby in the same room with her during the night. If the child is slightly older it may be necessary to sit up with him all night and in this event the mother and father would ideally take shifts. Additionally, and of importance, is the need to advise on the avoidance of overheating that very night as already outlined in Chapter 3.

Prevention of Colds

Vitamin C

Many years ago it was postulated that large doses of ascorbic acid would prevent colds, but the evidence does not corroborate the postulate (*British Medical Journal* Leading Article 1976, Watson 1982).

Breast Feeding

Breast feeding has been shown to have a protective effect against respiratory illness (Cunningham 1977, Stott and West 1981) and more specifically against respiratory syncytial viral infection (Downham *et al*. 1976, Pullan *et al*. 1980), but Taylor *et al*. (1982) have questioned these conclusions by showing that an apparently reduced incidence of respiratory illness in relation to breast feeding is negated when allowance is also made for other influences, e.g. maternal smoking, low social status, overcrowding, poor care given to the child, and low birth weight. As such, the very fact that a child *is* breast fed implies a reverse of these influences, and that the absence of the adverse influences is the preventive factor.

PERSISTENT COUGH IN CHILDREN

The borderline between the persistent cough and the recurrent cough is often ill-defined, and the possible causes are considered together. While pertussis is the best-known cause, the commonest causes are unrecognized asthma and rapidly recurring viral infections. A cough tends to be considered persistent if it has continued for more than two weeks. In children with a persistent cough, chest X-ray is rarely necessary and rarely shows any abnormality. Management is dependent upon cause, and it will become evident that antibiotic use purely on the grounds of persistence is a pointless exercise.

Pertussis

Paroxysms of cough are the characteristic feature and develop one or two weeks after the start of the illness, which is initially indistinguishable from any other simple respiratory illness. The paroxysmal stage of the illness subsides gradually but the cough may continue for as long as 12 weeks and sometimes longer. The child should be quarantined and kept away from school for four weeks. It is uncommon to isolate the causative organism after this length of time, and Roberts and Williams (1981) found that newborn babies isolated from their siblings for safety (e.g. with grandmother) did not develop whooping cough if away for at least four weeks.

Antibiotic Use

Antibiotics have a place in prophylaxis, in aborting the disease during its early stages, in reducing infectivity of the established disease and in treating complicating chest infections.

Prophylaxis

The concept of giving prophylactic antibiotic to infants in contact with whooping cough was suggested by Arneil and McAllister (1977). Subsequently Trollfors and Rabo (1981) demonstrated the prophylactic value of erythromycin in six infants who escaped infection despite exposure from infected parents. A 14 day course is recommended, and Bass (1985) strongly advocates use of the estolate rather than the stearate for all spheres of pertussis prevention.

Patients justifying prophylaxis are infants under the age of three months who have yet to be immunized and those over the age of three months in whom the pertussis vaccine has been omitted. There is also justification for prophylaxis in non-immunized children of any age and in adults irrespective of their immune status. Adults can both suffer from the disease and act as a source of infection, and prior infection or immunization as a child does not necessarily prevent re-infection when adult (Trollfors and Rabo 1981).

Aborting the Disease

The place of erythromycin in aborting whooping cough, when given at the early undiagnosed 'cold and cough' stage is discussed previously in the section on the acute cough.

Reducing Infectivity

In the established disease, erythromycin is effective in reducing the length of time during which positive cultures are obtained, but does not alter the course of the disease (Islur *et al*. 1975).

Treating Complicating Chest Infection

Pneumonia will often be associated with collapse, and management of children will invariably take place in hospital.

The Use of Steroids in Pertussis

There is a natural reluctance to use steroids for any reason at any age, but is this over-cautious approach justified? The problems of adrenal suppression and osteoporosis relate to prolonged use and are not relevant to the short course, and the risk of enhanced activity in a duodenal ulcer or recrudescence of old tuberculosis has no relevance to the child. The short steroid course is used without much concern in patients of all ages with asthma, including older infants with wheezy bronchitis, but the course is usually brief and as a precaution is tailed off slowly. Is there any reason, therefore, why steroids should not be used in the severer instances of whooping cough? The use of a short steroid course in infants and small children, at an initial dose of 5 mg three times a day, caused a marked reduction in the number of spasms and a reduction in the overall duration of the cough, and is recommended by Zoumboulakis *et al.* (1973), Barrie (1982) and Dianese (1982).

Unrecognized Asthma

Over the age of two to three years, unrecognized asthma (cough variant asthma) is the commonest cause of a persistent cough. An example is a six-year-old girl whose cough had persisted for six weeks following a chest infection. Clinical examination was negative and peak flow readings were 100, 125 and 120 l/min (predicted level 185 l/min, Godfrey *et al.* 1970). An oral bronchodilator was given and four days later the cough had gone and peak flow readings were 150, 200 and 200 l/min. The mother was advised that the child had asthma (albeit mildly) and sodium cromoglycate by spinhaler was started. This child demonstrates the rapid and often dramatic disappearance of a persistent cough which follows the use of a bronchodilator, and the value to be gained by use of the mini-Wright peak flow meter.

Failure to recognize asthma as a cause of cough can result in a cough lasting for months or even years during which time the child may receive repeated courses of cough medicines, antihistamines and antibiotics, all of which have no influence.

Despite the absence of audible wheeze, clinical diagnosis is often possible. Just as the manifest asthmatic child will wheeze on exertion and in cold air, so the milder asthmatic child will *cough* on exertion and in cold air, and will usually cough at night. The cough is non-productive, and may develop *de-novo*, but will often date from a respiratory viral infection or a chest infection. About a third will have a story of associated atopy (eczema, hay fever, food allergy, allergic rhinitis) and about a third a family history of either asthma or atopy (Hannaway and Hopper 1982). These authors comment that auscultation on forced expiration may produce a prolonged expiration with a subtle expiratory wheeze. This finding is a valuable clinical sign in the diagnosis of unrecognized asthma and is worth looking for specifically, and can often be recognized by the naked ear at the end of the forced expiration needed to operate the mini-Wright peak flow meter. Levy and Bell (1984) additionally describe sleep disturbances as occurring in a third of children subsequently recognized as having asthma.

A suggestion that preventive therapy is hardly ever necessary in children with unrecognized asthma is probably wrong. Many of these children have exercise restriction which may not be recognized unless enquired about.

The cough caused by unrecognized asthma tends to occur in those over the age of three years because asthma presenting under this age is usually more severe and will usually therefore be manifest. It follows that a persistent cough in a child under this age is likely to have a different cause (see later), but the age of three years is not a rigid demarcation; some of Spelman's (1984) children were only two years old, and unusually, one child has been seen aged only ten months who presented with a three month persistent cough caused by unrecognized asthma.

The Allergic Cough

Unrecognized asthma is likely to be the mechanism underlying most instances of so-called allergic cough, but the post-nasal drip of allergic rhinitis may be a contributory factor.

Recurrent Colds and Coughs

Frequently recurring colds and coughs are seen mainly during the winter and occur predominantly in children under five, but most occur in those under three years of age. In the majority there is no obvious reason for their symptoms, and it is highly probable that the cause is rapidly recurring infection with different viral strains (Wilks 1973). Several different viruses can be present in the community at the same time, and Blair *et al.* (1970) identified eleven rhinoviruses belonging to seven different serotypes during a single winter among 31 children with respiratory illness.

It is clearly quite possible for a small child, immunologically susceptible to virus infections, to contract one infection after another in quick succession.

Management

In the great majority of children with recurrent colds and coughs there is neither specific treatment nor means of prevention, and the mother needs reassurance that her child is suffering from common infections and that there is no serious underlying disorder. Rarely it may be necessary to X-ray the chest for reassurance. Treatment is non-specific and antibiotics are used selectively.

In a minority, however, there could be an underlying disorder or circumstance and the following factors need consideration:

(1) *Cystic Fibrosis* The diagnosis is unlikely in a child who is otherwise well, and cystic fibrosis is more likely to cause recurring *chest infections* than simple colds and coughs. Consequent upon its rarity, it behoves the general practitioner to avoid causing unnecessary parental anxiety by too frequent referral for investigation (David and Phillips 1982).

(2) *Passive Smoking* Infants of mothers who smoke have significantly more admissions for bronchitis and pneumonia than infants of non-smoking mothers (Harlap and Davies 1974, Colley *et al.* 1974). If both parents smoke the risk of these infections is doubled. Passive smoking also increases the incidence of cough in children aged between eight and 19 years (Charlton 1984), and by inference would also affect younger children.

(3) *Gas Cooking* Children from homes in which gas is used for cooking have a higher incidence of respiratory symptoms and respiratory infection than children from homes where electricity is used (Melia *et al.* 1977).

(4) *Central Heating* It is not known whether the incidence or persistence of coughs is different in centrally heated houses as compared to houses without central heating, nor which ages might be affected if there is a difference. A general practice study would give the answer.

Rare Causes

Rare causes of a persistent cough in children include cystic fibrosis, tuberculosis, inhaled foreign body, a minor oesophagotracheal fistula and the psychogenic cough.

PERSISTENT COUGH IN ADULTS

In adults the emphasis is different. Chest X-ray *is* necessary and the overriding need is to exclude carcinoma of bronchus and tuberculosis although neither is a common cause of persistent cough.

Carcinoma of Bronchus

Cough is the most common early symptom, but presentation can also occur as haemoptysis, dyspnoea, pleuritic pain, unresolved pneumonia, upper limb pain, Horner's syndrome and metastatic symptoms. Absence of abnormal signs in the chest does not exclude the diagnosis.

Tuberculosis

All age groups need consideration, and the disease is possible in U.K. nationals as well as in immigrant populations. The patient typically exhibits cough, tiredness, anorexia, weight loss and sometimes haemoptysis. The incidence is higher in post-gastrectomy patients and those on steroids, and may unexpectedly be present in those with chronic bronchitis. Tuberculosis is increasingly a disease of the elderly, particularly men (Horne 1984).

Commoner Causes

Sinusitis and Rhinitis

Post-nasal drip has been quoted as the commonest cause of a persistent cough in adults, but with advances in knowledge, pride of place is now taken by unrecognized asthma.

Unrecognized Asthma

It is perhaps not widely recognized that asthma may appear for the first time at any age. The first awareness of asthma is usually a cough which persists beyond two weeks following a 'flu illness or chest infection. The patient will typically cough at night and on exertion; have an audible wheeze on forced expiration (despite a clear chest), and peak flow rates will be below predicted levels. Management follows the same lines as in children, and the use of a bronchodilator abolishes the cough. All are likely to need preventive therapy, e.g. beclomethasone.

The advent of asthma in middle-age has relevance to other medication. A β-blocker for example, would need replacement by an appropriate alternative.

Chronic Bronchitis and Bronchiectasis

Both are well-known causes of persistent or recurrent cough.

Hiatus Hernia

The regurgitation of gastric content to laryngeal and pharyngeal level triggers the cough.

Pertussis

Pertussis can be overlooked as a cause of persistent cough in adults, who have an illness very similar to children (Maclean 1982).

Uncommon Causes

These include carcinoma of larynx or trachea, metastatic tumours, sarcoidosis, pneumoconiosis and extrinsic allergic alevolitis.

Management and Antibiotic Use

Treatment is dependent upon cause. As distinct from the acute cough, the peristent cough *can* benefit from cough medicines. In carcinoma of the bronchus, particularly, cough suppressants are of value.

THE ABSENT COUGH

'Is there any other point to which you would wish to draw my attention?'
'To the curious incident of the dog in the night-time.'
'The dog did nothing in the night-time.'
'That was the curious incident,' remarked Sherlock Holmes.
('*Silver Blaze*', Arthur Conan Doyle)

The 'Flu-Like Illness

The absence of cough has three possible explanations. The patient might have influenza or a respiratory viral illness, but the cough has yet to appear. Secondly, the illness might be an enterovirus 'flu typified by the triad of pyrexia, headache and myalgia only, or thirdly, the patient might have a different diagnosis altogether (Chapter 14).

Pneumonia

The absence of cough does not exclude the diagnosis.

PUO in Children

It is the absence of both cold and cough which in most instances gives the doctor the knowledge that one of several possible diagnoses may emerge (Chapter 13).

Tonsillitis

In the context of arguing that tonsillitis has a combined viral and bacterial cause (Chapter 4), the absence of cough does not necessarily mean the absence of a virus, but is likely to indicate the *presence* of a non-respiratory virus, e.g. an enterovirus.

Croup

It has been suggested that the presence or absence of an 'upper' respiratory illness including cough may be used as a guide to distinguish between acute laryngo-tracheitis (with cough) and acute epiglottitis (without cough), but in fact the presence or absence of an 'upper' respiratory illness is an unreliable diagnostic index (Chapter 7).

REFERENCES

Arneil, G. C. and McAllister, T. A. (1977). Prevention of whooping cough by antibiotics. *The Practitioner*, **219**, 855–858

Barrie, H. (1982). Treatment of whooping cough. *Lancet*, **2**, 830–831

Bass, J. W. (1985). Erythromycin for pertussis: probable reasons for past failures. *Lancet*, **2**, 147

Blair, W., Brown, W. K., Clarke, A., Jubb, L. G., Primrose, D., Wilson, T. S., Grist, N. R., Landsman, J. B. and Stott, E. J. (1970). Clinical and virological investigations of acute respiratory disease in children outside hospital. *J. R. Coll. Gen. Pract.*, **20**, 27-31

Carpenter, R. G., Gardner, A., Pursall, E., McWeeny, P. M. and Emery, J. L. (1979). Identification of some infants at immediate risk of dying unexpectedly and justifying intensive study. *Lancet*, **2**, 343-346

Charlton, A. (1984). Children's coughs related to parental smoking. *Br. Med. J.*, **288**, 1647-1649

Colley, J. R. T., Holland, W. W. and Corkhill, R. T. (1974). Influence of passive smoking and parental phlegm on pneumonia and bronchitis in early childhood. *Lancet*, **2**, 1031-1034

Cunningham, A. S. (1977). Morbidity in breast-fed and artificially fed infants. *J. Pediatr.*, **90**, 726-729

David, T. J. and Phillips, B. M. (1982). Overdiagnosis of cystic fibrosis. *Lancet*, **2**, 1204-1205

Dianese, G. (1982). Treatment of whooping cough. *Lancet*, **2**, 1224-1225

Downham, M. A. P. S., Gardner, P. S., McQuillin, J. and Ferris, J. A. J. (1975). Role of respiratory viruses in child mortality. *Br. Med. J.*, **1**, 235-239

Downham, M A. P. S., Scott, R., Sims, D. G., Webb, J. K. G. and Gardner, P. S. (1976). Breast-feeding protects against respiratory syncytial virus infections. *Br. Med. J.*, **2**, 274-276

Epidemiology (1980). Epidemiology of *Mycoplasma pneumoniae* infection in the British Isles, 1974-9. *J. Infect.*, **2**, 191-194

Foy, H. J., Kenny, G. E., Cooney, M. K. and Allan, I. D. (1979). Long-term epidemiology of infections with *Mycoplasma pneumoniae*. *J. Infect. Dis.*, **139**, 681-687

Godfrey, S., Kamburoff, P. L. and Nairn, J. R. (1970). Spirometry, lung volumes and airway resistance in normal children aged 5-18 years. *Br. J. Dis. Chest*, **64**, 15-24

Hannaway, P. J. and Hopper, D. K. (1982). Cough variant asthma in children. *J. Am. Med. Assoc.*, **247**, 206-208

Harlap, S. and Davies, A. M. (1974). Infant admissions to hospital and maternal smoking. *Lancet*, **1**, 529-532

Herzog, Ch., Just, M., Berger, R., Havas, L. and Fernex, M. (1983). Intranasal interferon for contact prophylaxis against common cold in families. *Lancet*, **2**, 962

Higgins, P. G. (1974). Virus isolations from patients in general practice, 1961-71. *J. Hyg. Camb.*, **72**, 255-264

Horn, M. E. C., Brain, E. A., Gregg, I., Inglis, J. M., Yealland, S. J. and Taylor, P. (1979). Respiratory viral infection and wheezy bronchitis in childhood. *Thorax*, **34**, 23-28

Horne, N. W. (1984). Problems of tuberculosis in decline. *Br. Med. J.*, **288**, 1249-1251

Islur, J., Auglin, C. S. and Middleton, P. J. (1975). The whooping cough

syndrome: a continuing paediatric problem. *Clin. Paediatr.*, **14**, 171-176
Krech, U., Price, P.C. and Jung, M. (1976). The laboratory diagnosis and epidemiology of *Mycoplasma pneumoniae* in Switzerland. *Infection*, **4**, (Suppl.) 33-36
Leading Article (1976). Vitamin C and the common cold. *Br. Med. J.*, **1**, 606-607
Levy, M. and Bell, L. (1984). General practice audit of asthma in childhood. *Br. Med. J.*, **289**, 1115-1116
Lewis, H.M., Parry, J.V., Davies, H.A., Parry, R.P., Mott, A., Doursmashkin, R.R., Sanderson, P.J., Tyrrell, D.A.J. and Valman, H.B. (1979). A year's experience of the rotavirus syndrome and its association with respiratory illness. *Arch. Dis. Child.*, **54**, 339-346
Maclean, D.W. (1982). Adults with pertussis. *J. R. Coll. Gen. Pract.*, **32**, 298-300
McSherry, J.A. (1981). Why not prescribe antibiotics for "heavy colds"? *J. R. Coll. Gen. Pract.*, **31**, 49
Mardh, P.A., Hovelius, B., Nordenfelt, E., Rosenberg, R. and Soltesz, L.V. (1976). The incidence and aetiology of respiratory tract infections in general practice - with emphasis on *Mycoplasma pneumoniae*. *Infection*, **4** (Suppl.) 40-48
Martin, A.J., Gardner, P.S. and McQuillin, J. (1978). Epidemiology of respiratory viral infection among paediatric in-patients over a six year period in North East England. *Lancet*, **2**, 1035-1038
Melia, R.J.W., Florey, C.duV., Altman, D.G. and Swan, A.V. (1977). Association between gas cooking and respiratory disease in children. *Br. Med. J.*, **2**, 149-152
Moazam, F., Talbert, J.L. and Rodgers, B.M. (1983). Foreign bodies in the pediatric tracheobronchial tree. *Clin. Pediatr.*, **22**, 148-150
Noah, N.D. (1974). *Mycoplasma pneumoniae* infection in the United Kingdom - 1967-73. *Br. Med. J*, **2**, 544-546
Phillpotts, R.J., Jones, R.W., Delong, D.C., Reed, S.E., Wallace, J. and Tyrrell, D.A.J. (1981). The activity of enviroxime against rhinovirus infection in man. *Lancet*, **1**, 1342-1344
Poole, P.M. and Tobin, J.O'H. (1973). Viral and epidemiological findings in MRC/PHLS surveys of respiratory disease in hospital and general practice. *Postgrad. Med. J.*, **49**, 778-787
Pullan, C.R., Toms, G.L., Martin, A.J., Gardner, P.S., Webb, J.K.G. and Appleton, D.R. (1980). Breast-feeding and respiratory syncytial virus infection. *Br. Med. J.*, **281**, 1034-1036
Roberts, A. and Williams, W.O. (1981). Whooping cough in nursery school children. *J. R. Coll. Gen. Pract.*, **31**, 470-472
Spelman, R. (1984). Chronic or recurrent cough in children - a presentation of asthma? *J. R. Coll. Gen. Pract.*, **34**, 221-222
Stanton, A.N. (1984). Overheating and Cot Death. *Lancet*, **2**, 1199-1201

Stott, N. C. H. and West, R. R. (1976). Randomised controlled trial of antibiotics in patients with cough and purulent sputum. *Br. Med. J.*, **2**, 556–559

Stott, N. C. H. and West, R. R. (1981). Acute lower respiratory tract infections in infants: the influence of central heating systems. *J. R. Coll. Gen. Pract.*, **31**, 148–150

Taylor, B., Wadsworth, J., Golding, J. and Butler, N. (1982). Breast-feeding, bronchitis, and admissions for lower-respiratory illness and gastro-enteritis during the first five years. *Lancet*, **1**, 1227–1229

Trollfors, B. and Rabo, E. (1981). Whooping cough in adults. *Br. Med. J.*, **283**, 696–697

Watson, G. I. (1982). *Epidemiology and Research in a General Practice*, p. 76. (London: Royal College of General Practitioners)

Wilks, J. M. (1973). Acute viral respiratory infections in a general practice during 1971. *J. R. Coll. Gen. Pract.*, **23**, 776–782

Williams, A. L., Uren, E. C. and Bretherton, L. (1984). Respiratory viruses and sudden infant death. *Br. Med. J.*, **288**, 1491–1493

Zoumboulakis, D., Anagnostakis, D., Albanis, V. and Matsaniotis, N. (1973). Steroids in treatment of pertussis. *Arch. Dis. Child.*, **48**, 51

9
Wheezy Bronchitis in Children

The Nature of Wheezy Bronchitis - Recognition of Asthma - Management of the Acute Episode - Longer-term Management - Differential Diagnosis

Should antibiotics be given to children with wheezy bronchitis? The answer lies in an understanding of asthma.

THE NATURE OF WHEEZY BRONCHITIS

There is ample evidence that wheezy bronchitis is an attack of asthma occurring in an asthmatic child. It is easy to see how wheezy bronchitis could be mistaken for a bacterial infection because the child is often *apparently* well in between attacks. Exercise tests, however, undertaken while wheezy bronchitic children are well and in between attacks, demonstrate respiratory resistance (Lenney and Milner 1978).

The more severe forms of asthma appear for the first time when the child is very young, e.g. under 18 months old, and these children will subsequently have many episodes of wheezy bronchitis and will sometimes have evidence of manifest asthma in between episodes. The milder forms of asthma tend to appear for the first time in slightly older children who will have episodes of wheezy bronchitis less frequently, and these episodes may be the only obvious manifestation of asthma. In between attacks such children are apparently well.

An attack of asthma (status asthmaticus) may be triggered by allergen, exercise, emotion or viral infection. Clinically, the attack of asthma and the episode of wheezy bronchitis are the same, with the exception that cold and cough will usually accompany the latter. A suggestion that asthma and wheezy bronchitis are not the same disorder is refuted by Sibbald et al. (1980) who concluded that both share a common genetic defect, although the manifestation of asthma may be influenced by other factors, e.g. atopy, which is not essential for the development of wheezy bronchitis.

The viral trigger embraces a wide range of viruses (Horn et al. 1979a). Rhinoviruses are identified most often; para-influenza viruses, respiratory syncytial virus and enteroviruses less often, and those found least often are Influenza A, Influenza B, adenoviruses, and *Mycoplasma pneumoniae* (Horn et al. 1979b). Once a child has been infected with a particular viral strain, immunity to that strain develops, and this could explain why episodes of wheezy bronchitis become less frequent as the child gets older.

Conclusions

Two conclusions can be drawn. Firstly, wheezy bronchitis is an attack of asthma induced by a viral infection occurring in an asthmatic child. The second conclusion is more subtle. The realization that wheezy bronchitis is a manifestation of asthma emphasizes the need to recognize asthma in its various forms and so enable a more adequate management of the asthmatic child.

RECOGNITION OF ASTHMA

Both general practitioners and hospital medical staff have been criticized for underdiagnosis and undertreatment. The basis for the criticism is the doctors' pre-occupation with infection and a reluctance to use the word asthma. Avoidance of the word asthma has been a tradition designed to prevent parental anxiety, but there is now evidence that a reluctance to use the term leads to underdiagnosis which in turn ensures undertreatment and enhances parental anxiety (Speight et al. 1983). If the disease is labelled and brought out into the open, treatment is more effective and parents more contented (Lee et al. 1983). In particular, effective prevention and long-term management become possible.

The very useful community campaign against asthma (Colver 1984) was impressive in demonstrating the degree of learning that is still necessary. Many practices seemed unaware that asthma and wheezy bronchitis were similar, and there was considerable erroneous adherence to the view that unrecognized asthma did not exist.

The diagnosis of asthma is obvious in the child who wheezes in between episodes of wheezy bronchitis, but the child with milder asthma who tends not to wheeze in between episodes may escape recognition. Evidence for silent asthma will commonly be present but children are very adaptive and the evidence needs to be looked for. As already discussed in the section on unrecognized asthma (Chapter 8), some will have the persistent night cough and there may be evidence of sleep disturbance, but the particular feature to look for is evidence of exercise restriction, particularly in cold, dry air. One method of doing this is to demonstrate sub-optimal peak-flow readings after exertion and/or improved readings following trial bronchodilation, but simple questioning about what the child *cannot* do will often give the answer (Periera Gray 1983). Enquiry should be made about exercise ability in relation to games, running and walking to and from school etc. The most useful clinical sign of silent asthma is the slight wheeze audible through the stethoscope on forced expiration, or heard with the naked ear at the end of the forced expiration needed to operate the peak-flow meter.

MANAGEMENT OF THE ACUTE EPISODE
Bronchodilators and Steroids

Inhalers have no relevance to small children who cannot use them, and are of little value during an acute episode of asthma because the tightness of the breathing prevents much of the drug being inhaled, but the development of the spacer has offset this drawback to a certain extent (Freelander and van Asperen 1984, Cox *et al.* 1984, Lee and Evans 1984).

Milder episodes of wheezy bronchitis occurring particularly in the older child might occasionally be controlled by an oral bronchodilator alone, but nearly always something more is needed. The addition of a short steroid course will commonly be adequate although the time taken for significant effect may take some hours. Prednisolone needs to be given in adequate dosage, e.g. 10 mg immediately followed by 15 mg three times a day for about 48 hours, and only then, when the child is virtually 'better', is the dose tailed off over two or three days. This combination of bronchodilator and steroid is effective and widely used.

Of many available bronchodilator drugs, orciprenaline or salbutamol or terbutaline are most suitable. Theophylline is a further option but consideration is needed before prescribing it. Variations in absorption can result in swings from subtherapeutic to toxic levels on the same daily dose (Denning *et al.* 1984) and the use of intravenous aminophylline (Woodcock *et al.* 1983, Stewart *et al.* 1984), or erythromycin (Prince *et al.* 1981) in a patient already taking theophylline can result in theophylline toxicity. It is acknowledged that the availability of a nebulized bronchodilator could now obviate the need for intravenous aminophylline, and it is also acknowledged that antibiotics are not the treatment of choice, but in the general practice setting with night duty rotas, it is possible that an antibiotic, perhaps erythromycin, might be added to a bronchodilator regime during the evening or night.

During an acute episode of wheezy bronchitis, prevention inhalers, e.g. sodium cromoglycate are temporarily discontinued, and restarted again when the child has regained sufficient 'puff'.

Infants

Infants with wheezy bronchitis have long been a problem because the response to oral bronchodilators under the age of 18 months has been negligible. There is variation in the age at which bronchial wall smooth muscle develops and responds to bronchodilators, and these drugs are more effective when given by inhalation. In the more significant illness, therefore, a nebulized bronchodilator is the treatment of choice, even though there will be uncertainty of the response, and nebulized ipratopium bromide may be more effective than nebulized salbutamol in those under the age of 18 months (Hodges *et al.* 1981).

Oral bronchodilators are worth trying, e.g. definitively in the mild illness, or prior to or following nebulization in the more severe illness. Either salbutamol or terbutaline in reduced dosage may be used.

Nebulization

Nebulizers have an advantage because there is no requirement for active inhalation to be timed with delivery, and the constant availability of the drug ensures inhalation even though the tightness of the asthma initially precludes much respiratory excursion. A nebulized bronchodilator has application to all age groups but is of particular value in the severe episode and in the small child.

Salbutamol is most commonly used. A doctor may feel concern about the possibility of overdose but concern is unfounded. Crompton (1984) makes the point that the nebulized dose of salbutamol is far greater than that delivered by the inhaler, and the deaths in the 1960s which had been thought to be caused by overuse of a ventolin inhaler were likely, in fact, to have been caused by inadequate treatment of the asthma, i.e. delay in the use of steroids.

Suggested dose regimes vary, and the simplest is to use two salbutamol nebules of 2.5 mg each for adults nebulized over ten to 15 minutes, and one salbutamol nebule for a child, but the duration of administration in children might be shortened. Jenkinson (1984) makes the point that it is more useful to think in terms of minutes than in milligrams. Dosages in infants and small children are theoretically smaller, but a small child may not accept a face mask, and an adequate method of delivery is to blow the nebulized mist onto the face. As much is wasted, detailed dose reduction is irrelevant.

Adequate additional use of steroids is important because only a part of the airflow obstruction in wheezy bronchitis is reversed by bronchodilators (Horn *et al.* 1979b). The improvement achieved by nebulization can be followed subsequently by worsening, and this is particularly likely to occur during the night. Much depends upon clinical judgement, but broadly speaking if two successive administrations are necessary, or if the time between administrations is less than three hours then steroids should be given as well, and clinical judgement will again decide whether the child should be admitted to hospital.

This additional need for steroids has particular relevance to home nebulization. The dramatic improvement achieved can create a false sense of security, and parents may fail to seek advice sufficiently early for steroids to be readily effective. Lillington *et al.* (1983) cite several instances of small children given nebulized salbutamol at home and subsequently admitted with severe asthma, and one of these children died. Home nebulization in children with an acute attack of wheezy bronchitis should be under the constant guidance of the general practitioner (Jenkinson 1983).

Asthma Deaths

Both children and adults can still die from asthma and knowledge of this fact is half the battle. Severity is equated with duration of illness and a previous bad night and there should be no hesitation in admitting a child to hospital if progress is slow. It is better to over-use rather than under-use steroids, i.e. if uncertain, prescribe.

Asthma deaths are more common during the summer (Khot and Burn 1984). One explanation might be the raised Ascomycetes ascospore concentration (Davies and Mullins 1984), but possibly more significant is the holiday season. A great increase in the incidence of asthma at St. Ives, Cornwall, was attributed to an increased exposure to house dust in holiday accommodation, to emotional strain while away from home, and to usual drugs inadvertently being left at home (Whyte and Philip 1984). While advice can very usefully be given to families going on holiday (e.g. taking own pillow and freshly washed sleeping bag), another method of prevention is more fundamental. Once again, it can be argued that if asthma is openly labelled and trouble taken to recognize it, then a child already diagnosed and adequately managed in prevention terms will be less likely to have serious trouble in adverse circumstances.

Antibiotics

A 'chest full of signs' is an emotive indication for antibiotic prescribing, and even with recognition that wheezy bronchitis is an attack of asthma triggered by a viral infection, some doctors would still prefer to prescribe antibiotics. The particular point to make is that whether antibiotics are given or not, the definitive treatment is for asthma.

It can be theoretically argued that antibiotics should be given because the narrowing of the bronchi due to oedema and mucus will encourage secondary bacterial infection, but this argument cannot be wholly true because many children recover with asthma treatment alone. Shapiro *et al.* (1974) found no benefit from the use of antibiotics, nor complications resulting from their exclusion.

A further approach is to remember that wheezy bronchitis represents a viral infection, and that the guidelines of selective antibiotic use should apply. Occasionally otitis media or tonsillitis may be associated and some children *will* have a chest infection, but the overall incidence of pneumonia in wheezy bronchitis occurring in the community is very low. The particular problem in asthma is the difficulty in recognizing a chest infection, and it is important to listen to the chest again when the bronchospasm has eased. Other features of a chest infection will need consideration, e.g. pyrexia, chest pain, abdominal pain, and if there is uncertainty, of course an antibiotic is justified.

Gregg (1984) postulates that widespread antibiotic use might unwittingly be beneficial in preventing long-term bronchial damage, and suggests that the additional use of an antibiotic should not be criticized out of hand.

If an antibiotic is given, the drug chosen will depend upon the site of infection, i.e. ear, throat or chest. If a chest infection is thought to be present, a broad spectrum antibiotic, e.g. amoxycillin or co-trimoxazole would generally be used for children of all ages, but in the presence of frank pneumonia, erythromycin may be preferred for children over five years of age owing to the incidence of *Mycoplasma pneumoniae* as a cause of pneumonia (Chapter 10). As already emphasized, however, if the child is taking theophylline, either erythromycin should not be used or an alternative bronchodilator prescribed.

The question may be asked again, 'Should antibiotics be given to children with wheezy bronchitis?' One answer is to advocate selective antibiotic use but this advocacy does not really answer the question. The point at issue is whether antibiotics are necessary in the more common situation when a chest infection is *unlikely* to be present. Another answer, therefore, is to beg the question, and state that whether antibiotics are given or not, all require treatment for asthma. A third and more realistic answer is to give antibiotics if recovery is not progressing satisfactorily after 24–48 hours, but it has to be recognized that a continuance of bronchospasm might well represent inadequate asthma treatment rather than antibiotic need. Infrequently, a persistent wheezy bronchitis despite an apparently adequate asthma control might reflect infection by *Mycoplasma pneumoniae*, and the use of, or a change to erythromycin is worthwhile.

Antiviral Drugs

The finding by Horn *et al.* (1979b) that rhinoviruses were identified most often in wheezy bronchitis allows speculation that antiviral drugs might have a role in the future.

LONGER-TERM MANAGEMENT

Sodium Cromoglycate and Beclomethasone Dipropionate

The introduction of inhaled sodium cromoglycate some fifteen years ago revolutionized the management of asthma in children, and the subsequent appearance of inhaled beclomethasone gave similar benefit to adults. Sodium cromoglycate is less effective in adults, and a child who has asthma continuing into the teens will need a change-over to beclomethasone (preferably by rotahaler), sometimes as early as 10–12 years of age. The preventive nature of these agents needs emphasis because some patients have difficulty in understanding the difference between long-term prevention and short-term treatment. Detailed explanation may be necessary to ensure that preventive agents are used regularly every day, even when well.

Benefit from prevention may be expected by those with unrecognized asthma (Chapter 8) and also by those with infrequent episodes of wheezy bronchitis who are apparently well in between, as well as by those with frequent episodes and manifest asthma in between. Seasonal asthma (hay fever) can also benefit; inhalations are started in advance of the season and continued until its end. Advice on the frequency of spinhaler use needs commonsense. Four times a day may be necessary, but three times is more realistic because the second inhalation can be taken at tea-time when home from school. Twice daily is better than nothing and can be helpful.

Inhaled sodium cromoglycate is safe, and with relevance to older children particularly, the long-term use of inhaled beclomethasone in children is also safe and free from adrenal suppression in doses up to 400 μg/24 hours (Morrow-Brown and Storey 1973, Bhan *et al.* 1980). The whole philosophy of prevention is that the agent should be used regularly on a long-term basis, and in many instances this will preclude the need for bronchodilator drugs as well, but a bronchodilator should be kept in the house for occasional short-term use if and when necessary.

Small Children

Because small children are incapable of conscious inspiration and expiration, inhalers cannot be used until the age of 4–5 years, and one option is to treat each episode of wheezy bronchitis as it occurs, without any long-term prevention. Such management is often inadequate, and in severe instances regular nebulized sodium cromoglycate at home is justified, and was effective in two thirds of toddlers (Lewis and Lewis 1984). More often, however, a bronchodilator is given on a long-term basis and theophylline is most commonly used, but as already mentioned the risk of toxicity needs to be borne in mind owing to the variation in absorption, the interaction with erythromycin and the additive effect of intravenous aminophylline.

A drawback to the long-term use of theophylline in older children is an incidence of behavioural problems (Furukawa *et al.* 1984), and a change to sodium cromoglycate should be made as soon as the child is old enough to inhale.

Ketotifen

Ketotifen can be given orally to children down to the age of two years, and does exert a preventative effect in a dose of 1 mg twice daily, but takes from 8–12 weeks to achieve it. This delay coupled with the side effect of drowsiness in a small proportion of patients has precluded enthusiasm for its widespread use.

Steroids

The very bad asthmatic is rarely seen, and the resulting growth retardation, chest deformity and hyperinflation a thing of the past. Long-term oral steroids do have a place but are rarely necessary. In a difficult situation, a shorter steroid course, e.g. two weeks, can produce improvement and allow time to rethink management (Milner 1982). Sometimes repeated short or 'crash' courses are necessary. Ideal management in the severe asthmatic child would combine the regular long-term use of both beclomethasone *and* a bronchodilator, and the latter might be given with greater benefit by nebulization at home, but in practice, the degree of severity demanding this type of management occurs more often in teenagers and adults.

Allergen Avoidance and Desensitization

Laying Dust

Dust precautions failed to help adults with mild asthma, all of whom were skin-test positive to the house dust mite (Burr *et al.* 1976), but this does not necessarily mean that children or severe asthmatics would gain no benefit, and advice about laying dust is well worth giving. The child's mother is given an instruction sheet which emphasizes frequent damp dusting, vacuum cleaning, the avoidance of too much dust-collecting bric-a-brac, plastic mattress covers, and periodic curtain washing. Pillows should be 'non-allergic', i.e. neither feather nor flock. Lee (1984) recommends an open sprung or slatted bed base, washable rugs rather than a fitted carpet, and washable bedding of terylene or polyester/cotton mix. Nylon is unsuitable because it develops a static charge which holds dust particles. The avoidance of excessive dust exposure while on holiday has already been discussed in the context of asthma deaths. Blow central heating is unsatisfactory because it stirs up dust.

A new approach is to kill the house dust mite or the mould on which it feeds, and trials of relevant chemicals are taking place.

Pets

The family cat or dog may be the source of allergen. Fortunately, sodium cromoglycate or beclomethasone usually achieve adequate prevention despite retention of this allergen source, and obviate the need to lose what might be a 'member of the family'. Simple avoidance of the animal is inadequate because fur and dander adhere to furniture. Pets should not be allowed in the bedroom.

Desensitization

Although there is a placebo effect, desensitization does help, but those benefitting most are the majority of children with asthma of moderate severity (Warner *et al.* 1978, Price *et al.* 1984). Children with mild or severe asthma gain less benefit. For this reason, and owing to the competence of modern pharmaceutical methods of prevention, and owing to the rare but real risk of fatal anaphylaxis, there can now be no justification in recommending desensitization as a means of prevention. This view endorses the conclusion reached by Rands and Godfrey (1983), and incidentally applies with equal force to hay fever.

Natural History

When should preventive measures be discontinued? In a prospective study of children with asthma who were followed from the age of seven to 21 years, Martin *et al.* (1980) distinguished between infrequent and frequent wheeze in childhood. The former became wheeze-free in adolescence, but some still had occasional wheeze to the age of 21 years. Of the latter, most continued to wheeze through adolescence and into adulthood, but only a quarter had significant asthma as adults. Knowledge of natural history is invaluable in advising patients, but in practice some patients will discontinue preventive measures themselves as their degree of asthma clearly improves.

DIFFERENTIAL DIAGNOSIS

Not all children with an 'attack of asthma' will have wheezy bronchitis, but other causes are less common or rare. During the first year of life respiratory syncytial bronchiolitis may present a clinical picture consistent with wheezy bronchitis, and this is the only differential diagnosis which is seen with any degree of common-ness.

Rare causes include an inhaled foreign body, gastro-oesophageal reflux in infants, drugs, e.g. aspirin, and tumour or congenital abnormality causing narrowing of the trachea or bronchi.

REFERENCES

Bhan, G. L., Gwynn, C. M. and Morrison Smith, J. (1980). Growth and adrenal function of children on prolonged beclomethasone dipropionate treatment. *Lancet*, **1**, 96-97

Burr, M. L., St. Leger, A. S. and Neale, E. (1976). Anti-mite measures in mite-sensitive adult asthma. *Lancet*, **1**, 333-335

Colver, A. F. (1984). Community campaign against asthma. *Arch. Dis. Child.*, **59**, 449-452

Cox, I. D., Wallis, P. J. W. and Apps, M. C. P. (1984). Potential limitations of a conical spacer device in severe asthma. *Br. Med. J.*, **288**, 1044

Crompton, G. K. (1984). Illogical warnings on ventolin inhalers. *Br. Med. J.*, **288**, 1231-1232

Davies, B. H. and Mullins, J. (1984). Deaths from asthma. *Br. Med. J.*, **289**, 557

Denning, D. W., Cheriyan, G. and Tumwine, J. (1984). Further problems with theophylline. *Lancet*, **1**, 223

Freelander, M. and Van Asperen, P. P. (1984). Nebuhaler versus nebuliser in children with acute asthma. *Br. Med. J.*, **288**, 1873-1874

Furukawa, C. T., Shapiro, G. G., Du Hamel, T., Weimer, L., Pierson, W. E. and Bierman, C. W. (1984). Learning and behaviour problems associated with theophylline therapy. *Lancet*, **1**, 621

Gregg, I. (1984). Don't be alarmist about antibiotics and asthma. *Gen. Practit.*, June 29, 13

Hodges, I. G. C., Groggins, R. C., Milner, A. D. and Stokes, G. M. (1981). Bronchodilator effect of inhaled ipratropium bromide in wheezy toddlers. *Arch. Dis. Child.*, **56**, 729-732

Horn, M. E. C., Reed, S. E. and Taylor, P. (1979a). Role of viruses and bacteria in acute wheezy bronchitis in childhood: a study of sputum. *Arch. Dis. Child.*, **54**, 587-592

Horn, M. E. C., Brain, E. A., Gregg, I., Inglis, J. M., Yealland, S. J. and Taylor, P. (1979b). Respiratory viral infection and wheezy bronchitis in childhood. *Thorax*, **34**, 23-28

Jenkinson, D. (1983). Use of a nebulizer for acute asthma. *J. R. Coll. Gen. Pract.*, **33**, 725

Jenkinson, D. (1984). Personal communication

Khot, A. and Burn, R. (1984). Seasonal variation and trial trends of deaths from asthma in England and Wales 1960-82. *Br. Med. J.*, **289**, 233-234

Lee, D. A., Winslow, N. R., Speight, A. N. P. and Hey, E. N. (1983). Prevalence and spectrum of asthma in childhood. *Br. Med. J.*, **286**, 1256-1258

Lee, P. G. (1984). Allergy. *Second Opinion*, 1-16

Lee, H. and Evans, H. E. (1984). Aerosol bag for administration of bronchodilators to young asthmatic children. *Pediatrics*, **73**, 230-232

Lenney, W. and Milner, A. D. (1978). Recurrent wheezing in the pre-school child. *Arch. Dis. Child.*, **53**, 468-473

Lewis, G. M. and Lewis, R. A. (1984). The place of nebulisers in childhood asthma. *Maternal and Child Health*, **9**, 34-41

Lillington, A. W., Campbell, A. N. and Poulier, R. A. (1983). Safe drugs for childhood asthma? *Lancet*, **2**, 1032-1033

Martin, A. J., McLennan, L. A., Landau, L. I. and Phelan, P. D. (1980). The natural history of childhood asthma to adult life. *Br. Med. J.*, **280**, 1397-1400

Milner, A. D. (1982). Childhood asthma: treatment and severity. *Br. Med. J.*, **285**, 155-156

Morrow-Brown, H. and Storey, G. (1973). Beclomethasone dipropionate steroid aerosol in treatment of perennial allergic asthma in children. *Br. Med. J.*, **3**, 161-164

Periera Gray, D. J. (1983). Asthma in general practice. *Members' Reference Book*, Royal College of General Practitioners, 303-309

Price, J. F., Warner, J. O., Hey, E. N., Turner, M. W. and Soothill, J. F.

(1984). A controlled trial of hyposensitization with absorbed tyrosine *Dermatophagoides pteronyssinus* antigen in childhood asthma: *in vivo* aspects. *Clin. Allergy*, **14**, 209–219

Prince, R. A., Wing, D. S., Weinberger, M. M., Hendeles, L. S. and Riegelman, S. (1981). Effect of erythromycin on theophylline kinetics. *J. Allergy Clin. Immunol.*, **68**, 427–431

Rands, D. A. and Godfrey, R. C. (1983). Side effects of desensitization for allergy – a general practice survey. *J. R. Coll. Gen. Pract.*, **33**, 647–649

Shapiro, G. G., Eggleston, P. A., Pierson, W. E., Ray, C. G. and Bierman, C. W. (1974). Double-blind study of the effectiveness of a broad spectrum antibiotic in status asthmaticus. *Pediatrics*, **53**, 867–872

Sibbald, B., Horn, M. E. C. and Gregg, I. (1980). A family study of the genetic basis of asthma and wheezy bronchitis. *Arch. Dis. Child.*, **55**, 354–357

Speight, A. N. P., Lee, D. A. and Hey, E. N. (1983). Underdiagnosis and undertreatment of asthma in childhood. *Br. Med. J.*, **286**, 1253–1256

Stewart, M. F., Barclay, J. and Warburton, R. (1984). Risk of giving intravenous aminophylline to acutely ill patients receiving maintenance treatment with theophylline. *Br. Med. J.*, **288**, 450

Warner, J. O., Price, J. F., Soothill, J. F. and Hey, E. N. (1978). Controlled trial of hyposensitization to *Dermatophagoides pteronyssinus* in children with asthma. *Lancet*, **2**, 912–915

Woodcock, A. A., Johnson, M. A. and Geddes, D. M. (1983). Theophylline prescribing serum concentrations, and toxicity. *Lancet*, **2**, 610–612

Whyte, B. and Philip, C. J. (1984). Deaths from asthma. *Br. Med. J.*, **289**, 557

10
Pneumonia

Clinical Diagnosis – Investigation – Infective Causes – Management and Antibiotic Use – Differential Diagnosis

In making a clinical diagnosis the many and varied presentations need to be borne in mind. An early chest X-ray can be of value in proving or disproving the *presence* of pneumonia, but identification of infective cause requires additional investigation and is not established until later. Both hospital physicians and general practitioners are therefore obliged to initiate antibiotic treatment blind, and a rational choice has to depend upon a pre-existing knowledge of possible causes, their likely incidence, and their antibiotic susceptibility. This pre-existing knowledge coupled with an awareness of illness course is the cornerstone of intelligent general practice management because the exigencies of general practice may sometimes preclude all investigation.

CLINICAL DIAGNOSIS
Adults and Children

The classical presentation of high temperature, pleuritic pain, and cough is not common. More often, the patient presents with what appears to be an 'upper' respiratory illness or an influenzal illness. Two pyrexial patterns are recognizable, occurring with equal frequency and embracing all age groups, but having no significance in relation to infective cause. In one pattern the pyrexia and chest signs are present from early in the illness, and in the other (late pyrexia pattern) the pyrexia and chest signs develop after a prodromal phase of cold and/or cough. These are the pyrexial patterns which occur in uncomplicated 'upper' respiratory illness or ' 'flu', but *this* time the advent of pyrexia (late pyrexia pattern) *does* mean a chest infection rather than simply reflecting a normal pattern of illness.

Similarly, there are two patterns of cough. In one pattern the cough is present from the start of the illness and in the other the onset is delayed. A worsening cough might indicate the development of a chest infection, but the delayed onset of cough could represent either a chest infection or the uncomplicated illness pattern.

Two further pyrexial patterns are very suggestive. In a patient with ' 'flu', persistence of pyrexia beyond the expected time (e.g. more than three days) or a recrudescence of temperature after initial subsidence are both very likely to be caused by pneumonia. Similarly, in a child with a cold and cough, a persisting high temperature into the second or third day is very suggestive of a secondary bacterial infection which may be pneumonia. Pleuritic pain, non-pleuritic chest pain, unilateral abdominal pain or flank pain will sometimes occur and can be a guide to the diagnosis.

Patients with severe pneumonia, characterized by extreme dyspnoea, cyanosis, shock and multi-system disturbance are rarely seen by an individual general practitioner.

Variations in Presentation

PUO

Both adults and children will occasionally present in this way.

Predominant Pleuritic Pain

Usually occurring in adults, pneumonia is the cause in only a small proportion of patients (see Differential Diagnosis).

Absence of Pyrexia

About a third of patients (all ages) do not have a high temperature and give the impression of being apyrexial. The acute illness tends to be represented by chest pain, feeling unwell, dyspnoea or worsening cough, and in children sometimes by nothing more than sleepiness or being miserable or vomiting.

Absence of Cough

About one out of every six patients with pneumonia has no cough. Half will subsequently develop a cough but the remainder will have no cough throughout the illness. This phenomenon occurs in both adults and children, and is unrelated to any particular infective cause.

Absence of Illness

It can be disconcerting to have watched a child walk into the surgery, seemingly well, and to then find chest signs indicative of pneumonia, with subsequent radiological confirmation. This phenomenon is not common, but more than once a mother has commented on the paradox that her child was much more ill when having a seemingly 'milder' illness, e.g. ' 'flu'.

Physical Signs

What is heard will depend upon the stage of the illness. In practice, bronchial breathing is rarely heard, and by far the commonest abnormal physical sign is the presence of localized crepitations, sometimes accompanied by rhonchi or reduced breath sounds. Rhonchi may occasionally be the only abnormal finding. Possibly least recognized as having significance is the absence or reduction of breath sounds. This finding is sometimes the only abnormal physical sign and may easily be overlooked. A pleural rub is only occasionally heard. Roughly one out of every eight patients with pneumonia (adults and children) will have no abnormal signs at all. About half will subsequently develop signs, but the remainder will have a clear chest throughout the illness. The technique of ausculatory percussion (Guarino 1980) might be of use in this context.

The Elderly

The elderly exhibit features not seen in other age groups. The presentation of pneumonia can be relatively silent – silent until the chest is examined. In patients over the age of 80 years particularly, mental confusion may be the sole presenting feature. Acute confusion has several causes and two of the commonest are silent pneumonia and a silent urinary tract infection. Congestive cardiac failure may be the presenting feature but is not often seen because many elderly patients are already taking diuretics. When LVF is the presenting feature, the immediate chest signs obviate definitive diagnosis, and it is necessary to listen to the chest again after treatment of the failure. A cerebrovascular accident may be triggered by pneumonia. Evaluation of clinical signs in the elderly can be difficult because some patients have a few basal crepitations as a permanent and 'normal' feature. Chest X-ray is helpful.

Infants

In general practice the infant with a major chest infection is more likely to have respiratory syncytial viral bronchiolitis than pneumonia from any cause. Clinical features include a rapid respiratory rate, intercostal recession, flaring of the alae nasi, cough, fever, tachycardia, restlessness, and rarely the grunting respiration caused by pleural pain. Chest signs may be absent. Bronchospasm is more suggestive of bronchiolitis.

The clinical presentation of pneumonia may be non-specific, e.g. pyrexia with or without vomiting, or vomiting and diarrhoea. Diarrhoea occurring in infants and small children should be looked upon as 'symptom query cause' (Jolly 1984). Many *will* have gastroenteritis but other infective causes are possible including pneumonia.

INVESTIGATION

Early Chest X-ray

The main purpose of an early chest X-ray is to demonstrate the presence or absence of pneumonia, and with the exception of a rarely demonstrated abscess cavity (staphylococcal or Gram-negative or anaerobic aspiration pneumonia), is no guide to infective cause. Early chest X-ray is therefore instrumental in making the diagnosis in patients with PUO and in those with limited or absent physical signs. Conversely, as many as a third of patients clinically thought to have pneumonia have a clear chest on X-ray ('Not Pneumonia' – see later). X-ray may also demonstrate unexpected disorders which have relevance to management, e.g. cardiac failure, collapse, tuberculosis, secondary carcinoma.

The traditional distinction between lobar and segmental pneumonia on the one hand, and bronchopneumonia on the other serves no useful purpose.

Establishing Infective Cause

Sputum Culture

Sputum culture is a disappointing method of investigation, but better results can be achieved with sputum obtained by invasive techniques in hospital, e.g. transtracheal aspiration, bronchoscopic aspiration and direct lung puncture.

White Blood Count and Plasma Viscosity

Plasma viscosity is raised in most instances of pneumonia, but a raised white count with a leukocytosis is present in only half. A normal count does not therefore exclude pneumonia. The presence or absence of a raised white count is no reliable guide to infective cause.

Blood Culture

Bacteraemia occurs predominantly in pneumococcal pneumonia, and Macfarlane *et al*. (1982) recorded a 14% incidence.

Cold Agglutinins

Cold agglutinins are not found in every patient with *Mycoplasma pneumoniae* pneumonia and Macfarlane *et al*. (1982) have demonstrated their presence in pneumonia due to other causes including *Streptococcus pneumoniae*.

Detection of Pneumococcal Antigen

Using counter-current immunoelectrophoresis (CIE) Macfarlane *et al.* (1982) demonstrated that the detection of pneumococcal antigen in sputum particularly is a most effective method of identifying pneumococcal infection.

Serology

The demonstration of a four-fold or greater rise in titre on paired sera can identify several infective agents including *M. pneumoniae, Chlamydia psittaci, Coxiella burnetii, Legionella pneumophila*, and also viruses including Influenza A, Influenza B, adenoviruses, respiratory syncytial virus and para-influenza viruses. The first sample is taken during the first five days of the illness, and the second about two weeks after the illness starts. If it is too late to obtain an acute serum, a high titre in a single convalescent serum can suggest recent infection, and confirmation can sometimes be made by demonstrating a rise in the specific immunoglobulin titre.

Throat Swab for Viruses

Throat swab additionally enables identification of viral type or strain, and rhinoviruses and enteroviruses are usually identified by swab alone, but the method is disappointing and the pick-up rate low.

Immuno-Fluorescence

Respiratory syncytial virus can be rapidly identified by immuno-fluorescence of naso-pharyngeal aspirate, and this method is of greater use than serology in infants.

Investigation in General Practice

In practical terms, the two investigations of greatest value to the general practitioner are domiciliary chest X-ray and serology. The former confirms the presence or absence of pneumonia and may furnish other information, and the latter identifies several of the less common causes. This methodology reasonably assumes a negative serology to indicate pneumococcal pneumonia.

Because initial treatment is based upon pre-existing knowledge of cause and incidence, because this data tends to have been obtained from hospital studies, and because the incidence of causes in hospital and in general practice is different (see later), then investigation in the general practice setting has particular value. Unless studies *are* conducted in general practice, the true picture of cause and incidence will not be learned.

INFECTIVE CAUSES

Hospital physicians and general practitioners have a different view of pneumonia because the less severe instances tend to stay at home, whereas those more severely ill go to hospital. Table 10.1 demonstrates the recorded incidence of infective cause in three recent English studies. The incidence of identified cause is proportional to the extent and sophistication of investigation.

Streptococcus Pneumoniae

Incidence

The demonstration by Macfarlane *et al.* (1982) of a 76% incidence among adults with community-acquired pneumonia confirms the long-held belief that the pneumococcus is the commonest cause. The picture in general practice is less clear, but a two third incidence of negative serology (Table 10.1) suggests the same. In children over five years of age, *Mycoplasma pneumoniae* causes up to 20%, but the remainder are probably pneumococcal. Under five years, the incidence is high, being shared between *Haemophilus influenzae* and *Streptococcus pneumoniae* (Shann *et al.* 1984) and these two organisms most commonly cause the rare pneumonia complicating measles and pertussis. The pneumococcus is the commonest cause among elderly patients, and the pneumonia complicating Influenza A infection is more often pneumococcal than staphylococcal.

Distinctive Features

There are no reliably distinctive features; the classical presentation can be mimicked by other causes. Bacteraemic pneumococcal pneumonia is associated with greater severity of illness, sometimes shock, sometimes rigors, and a slower response to therapy, but there may be delay in clinical recognition of up to 72 hours (Dorff *et al.* 1973, Fenton *et al.* 1983). The possibility that the illness might worsen owing to bacteraemia should be borne in mind.

Mycoplasma Pneumoniae

Incidence

M. pneumoniae is likely to be the second commonest cause in general

	Nottingham Macfarlane et al. (1982) Hospital (Adults 127)	Bristol White et al. (1981) Hospital (Adults 210)	Plymouth Everett (1983) General practice (Adults 81) (Children 25)
Patients investigated			
Serology	126	106	69 { 4 children / 65 adults
Viral throat swab	113	10	28
Blood culture	127	128	
Culture sputum (Spontaneous)	77 ⎫	133	
Culture sputum (Tracheal saline)	42 ⎭ 119		
Culture tracheal aspirate	5		
Culture percutaneous lung aspirate	3		
Pneumococcal antigen (CIE)			
Blood	123		
Sputum	111		
Pleural fluid	18		
Concentrated urine	98		
Causes (%)			
Bacterial			
Pneumococcus	76.0	11.5	
Legionella pneumophila	15.0	1.5	
Staphylococcus aureus	2.4	4.0	
Haemophilus influenzae	3.0	2.0	
Other	0.8	2.0	
'Atypical'			
Mycoplasma pneumoniae	2.4	14.0	15.4
Chlamydia psittaci	5.5	1.5	4.6
Coxiella burnetii	0.8	3.0	

Table 10.1 Incidence of infective causes in patients with community-acquired and radiologically confirmed pneumonia in three English studies CIE = Counter-current immunoelectrophoresis. RSV = Respiratory syncytial virus

	Nottingham Macfarlane et al. (1982) Hospital (Adults 127)	Bristol White et al. (1981) Hospital (Adults 210)	Plymouth Everett (1983) General practice (Adults 81) (Children 25)
Virus			
Influenza A	4.7	10.5	4.6
Influenza B	0.8	2.0	
RSV	1.5	1.5	
Adenovirus	0.8		
Parinfluenza virus		1.0	
Varicella	0.8		
Measles			1.0
No Identifiable Pathogen	3.0	52.0	67.8
Other Causes (e.g. carcinoma, tuberculosis)	excluded from study	excluded from study	6.5

practice (Table 10.1). Foy *et al.* (1970) found that 20% of all investigated pneumonia in a five-year study had this cause, and established that the highest overall incidence occurred in children and teenagers aged between five and 19 years. The highest incidence of all was in the 5-9 year age group.

M. pneumoniae has not been considered to be a common cause, and low recorded instances may be explained because studies of pneumonia tend to be confined to adults. Another reason could be that studies are usually undertaken in hospital; it is probable that most instances of *M. pneumoniae* pneumonia are not severe and are managed at home. A further reason in general practice is that cases are missed and recover spontaneously while receiving the 'wrong' antibiotic, e.g. amoxycillin. There is factual evidence for such occurrences.

Distinctive Features

There are two misconceptions. Firstly, despite 'characteristic features' which are frequently described, there are in fact no distinctive features which enable a clinical diagnosis in the individual patient. The clinical features can mimic pneumococcal pneumonia in all respects, and most have lobar or segmental consolidation radiologically. The other misconception relates to the 'atypical' nature of the pneumonia, i.e. radiological findings in excess of physical signs. This phenomenon must occur because it is stated so often, but has not been seen in general practice.

The reason for both these misconceptions is possibly that *Mycoplasma pneumoniae* has not been adequately studied in the general practice setting, and emphasizes the argument already put forward for the general practice investigation of pneumonia.

Legionella Pneumophila

Incidence

The true incidence is uncertain. Macfarlane *et al.* (1982) demonstrated legionella pneumonia as the second commonest cause among 127 adults in hospital with community-acquired pneumonia, and the incidence is appreciable among those with hospital acquired pneumonia (Yu *et al.* 1982), but whether legionella pneumonia is also common in the community is more open to question. If milder cases are being missed and recovering spontaneously on the 'wrong' antibiotic, there should be evidence for a wide range of illness severity, but present evidence for the existence of milder illnesses is limited. If legionella pneumonia is occurring in general practice it is curious that serological testing has not yet identified it. Even though *Legionella pneumophila* may be the second commonest cause of pneumonia managed in hospital, it is likely that the second commonest cause in general practice is *M. pneumoniae*.

Distinctive Features

The general practitioner's guide to hospital admission would be one or more of the features of any severe pneumonia, i.e. a persisting high temperature, cyanosis, marked dyspnoea, mental confusion and hypotension. Legionella pneumonia can exhibit a multisystem disturbance including neurological abnormality and biochemical upset. Epidemiological factors might give a guide. Legionnaire's disease can be contracted in the United Kingdom, but a third of cases are associated with foreign travel. The occurrence of the disease in

America is well known, and Fallon (1983) records instances from Mediterranean holiday resorts; Spain, Portugal, Corfu, Italy and Majorca. Water is the source of infection, which may arise in mud, cooling towers, shower heads, air-conditioning units, and piped supplies and taps in hospitals and hotels.

Chlamydia Psittaci

Incidence

Psittacosis is not one of those rare diseases which 'only happen in hospital'. The incidence of 5% or less is similar in both hospital and general practice. The cases seen by one general practitioner in Plymouth during the last decade have occurred in an incidence of about one a year, and half have had a 'flu-like illness without chest infection and half pneumonia. This incidence is comparable to the occurrence of 18 symptomatic cases in one practice during an 8½ year period (Nagington 1984). Both adults and older children are affected.

Distinctive Features

There are no reliably distinctive features, and radiologically there may be segmental or lobar consolidation. Hospital physicians tend to look upon psittacosis pneumonia as a severe illness with a poor prognosis, because the severer illnesses go to hospital, but the patients seen in general practice have been no more ill than other patients with pneumonia managed at home, although the illnesses have been slightly more prolonged. Once again, the widely believed 'atypical' nature of psittacosis pneumonia has not been seen; chest signs have been manifest and have not been minimal in relation to radiological findings.

A psittacine association may suggest the diagnosis. Infection can arise from inhaling the secretions or dried excreta of a variety of infected birds, and relevant occupations include farming, veterinary work, pet shops, fish handling (gulls), and the chicken, turkey and duck processing industries. A psittacine association, however, is commonly absent. In the Cambridgeshire survey from 1975-83, only 17% of illnesses had an evident presumptive bird source, and this low figure coupled with an absence of seasonal variation implied endemicity (Nagington 1984). It is possible that animals, e.g. cats and dogs, may spread the disease from bird to man, and Nagington (1984) suggests that human to human spread may be more common than realized; a suggestion supported by Pether *et al.* (1984) and Isaacs (1984).

Coxiella Burnetii

Incidence

In all studies of pneumonia, the incidence of Q-fever is low; often less than 1%.

Distinctive Features

The diagnosis may be difficult. Presentation can occur as a 'flu-like illness with cough and pleuritic pain, but two patients (Ellis and Dunbar 1982) exhibited meningism without respiratory features and *did* have minimal chest signs despite radiological evidence of consolidation. Severe headache is a common feature (Salmon *et al.* 1982). The clinical features can include myocarditis, meningo-encephalitis, epididymo-orchitis, uveitis and hepatitis. Endocarditis occurs in about a fifth of those infected.

The diagnosis may be suggested by occupation. Cattle and sheep represent the reservoir of infection in Britain, and the disease may be contracted abroad. Relevant occupations embrace farms, slaughter houses, hides, fleeces and veterinary work. A further source of Q-fever is the American dog tick (*Dermacentor variabilis*) which is common in S.W. Nova Scotia and acts as a reservoir of *Coxiella burnetti* (Marrie *et al.* 1981).

Staphylococcus Aureus

Incidence and Distinctive Features

Staphylococcal pneumonia is a severe illness with an appreciable mortality, and patients presenting in general practice become more ill than usual with the features of a severe pneumonia, i.e. persisting high temperature, vomiting, mental confusion, hypotension, cyanosis and marked dyspnoea. These patients are admitted, and for this reason the incidence of staphylococcal pneumonia is virtually confined to hospital. A lung abscess may be seen on X-ray.

Staphylococcal pneumonia may complicate cystic fibrosis; has a higher incidence in diabetics than non-diabetics, and can occur in the whole age range from infancy to old age. Staphylococcal skin sepsis may be the initial cause in infants. The pneumonia complicating chicken pox in children is usually staphylococcal, but this organism is an infrequent cause of pneumonia complicating measles or pertussis. Despite classical teaching, the pneumonia complicating Influenza A is more often pneumococcal than staphylococcal.

Haemophilus Influenzae
Incidence and Distinctive Features

In infants and children under the age of five years, *H. influenzae* occurring alone or in conjunction with *Str. pneumoniae* is a common cause of pneumonia. The incidence of *H. influenzae* pneumonia in older children is uncertain, but is probably low, and in adults also the incidence is small (Table 10.1). When occurring in adults, *H. influenzae* pneumonia tends to arise in the elderly and in those with chronic obstructive airways disease. There are no distinctive features, but age and the described disease associations can be suggestive.

Viruses

A general practitioner could be forgiven for wondering whether viral pneumonia exists. Viral pneumonia is rare, fulminating and often fatal. The influenza and adenoviruses are more commonly the cause (Dhillon and Collins 1983), producing severe dyspnoea and hypoxia with few, if any, physical signs but extensive X-ray shadowing. It is problematical whether milder instances of viral pneumonia occur.

Despite the apparent rarity of viral pneumonia, viruses are likely to be widely implicated in the causation of pneumonia, but in the role of precursor to secondary bacterial infection rather than as a primary invader. The classic example is the bacterial pneumonia complicating Influenza A infection in adults, but a wide range of viruses have been found in association with pneumonia in all age groups from infancy to old age (Foy *et al.* 1970, Horn *et al.* 1975, Communicable Disease Report 1983a and 1983b, Shann *et al.* 1984). In general practice, for example, a patient has been seen with radiologically confirmed pneumonia complicating a rhinovirus 'flu-like illness. A common association between viruses and pneumonia is also suggested by the clinical presentations of pneumonia, which often reflect secondary bacterial infection occurring in 'upper' respiratory illness or ' 'flu'. That the actual 'pick-up' rate of viruses is low does not detract from the likelihood of their involvement.

Measles

The complicating pneumonia is invariably bacterial, and caused by a mixed flora, of which *Str. pneumoniae* and *H. influenzae* are most common. Staphylococci and streptococci are less common. The rare viral pneumonia is more prevalent in immuno-deficient children, e.g. those with protein malnutrition in less developed countries.

Chicken Pox

The viral pneumonia found typically in adults varies greatly in severity. Pneumonia in children is usually a secondary staphylococcal infection.

Other Causes

Other causes are rarely seen in general practice owing either to rarity itself, or because the pneumonia tends to be hospital-acquired.

Pertussis pneumonia has a similar bacteriology to measles pneumonia. Streptococcal pneumonia is now very rare; there is destruction of lung tissue and the illness is complicated by pleural effusion and empyema. Tuberculous pneumonia occurs particularly in the elderly, the very young and in those immunologically compromised; the illness resembles acute bacterial pneumonia. Aspiration pneumonia can be associated with dental sepsis, and may be secondary to oesophageal obstruction or loss of consciousness; bacteriology is predominantly mixed aerobic and anaerobic. Lipoid pneumonia is caused by the regular ingestion of liquid paraffin in elderly people with oesophageal reflux and diminished cough reflex, and may cause an apparent unresolved pneumonia (Rachappa *et al.* 1984). The demonstration of lipophages in the sputum confirms the diagnosis. Gram-negative pneumonia caused by *Klebsiella spp., Pseudomonas spp.*, enterobacter or *E. coli* occurs at any age and is more prevalent in patients with serious underlying disease, e.g. chronic lung disease, neoplasia, alcoholism, diabetes and in those immunosuppressed. Antecedent antibiotic use may also be a contributory factor. *Chlamydia trachomatis* is a rare cause in infants (Beem and Saxon 1977) and can develop after delivery through chlamydia-infected cervices (Schachter *et al.* 1979).

Immuno-suppression may be caused by steroids, immunosuppressive drugs, or disease, e.g. leukaemia, lymphoma, myelomatosis, acquired immune deficiency syndrome (AIDS), and may follow splenectomy or be hereditary. Pneumonia may be caused by a wide variety of agents occurring singly or in improbable combinations (Dhillon and Collins 1983), including fungi, cytomegalovirus and *Pneumocystis carinii*.

MANAGEMENT AND ANTIBIOTIC USE

Home Management

Home management demands reasonably adequate home conditions and the presence of a responsible person in the house, both to care for the patient and to seek advice should this be necessary. These criteria should be adhered to rigidly. The doctor should visit daily in the early stages of the illness, and will watch for any immediate worsening (e.g. staphylococcal or bacteraemic pneumococcal pneumonia); will see that cardiac failure is adequately treated, and will watch for any antibiotic side effects, e.g. diarrhoea, which would indicate an antibiotic change over and above the dictates of the illness itself.

Initial Antibiotic Choice

Infants and those with a severe pneumonia are admitted to hospital. Of adults and children suitable for home management, the four infective causes of pneumonia which need consideration are *Str. pneumoniae, M. pneumoniae, Chlamydia psittaci* and *H. influenzae*. Three further causes; *Staphylococcus aureus, Legionella pneumophila*, and *Coxiella burnetii* (Q-fever) may be borne in mind but are possibly less relevant.

Penicillin

Although pneumococcal strains with resistance to penicillin have been reported in South Africa (Jacobs and Koornhof 1978) and Papua New

Guinea (Gratten *et al.* 1980), pneumococcal pneumonia can still be adequately treated with penicillin in most countries, but amoxycillin or ampicillin are better initial choices because these two antibiotics are also effective against *H. influenzae*.

Amoxycillin or Ampicillin

Amoxycillin has been considered preferable to ampicillin owing to a slightly better absorption and a lower diarrhoea potential. The initial use of amoxycillin is suitable for children under five years of age because *Str. pneumoniae* and *H. influenzae* are the commoner causes, and for adults of any age because a majority will have pneumococcal pneumonia, but amoxycillin is ineffective against *M. pneumoniae, Chlamydia psittaci, Legionella pneumophila, Staphylococcus aureus* and *Coxiella burnetii*, and a subsequent change to a more appropriate antibiotic may become necessary in some patients. Amoxycillin is used in adequate dosage, e.g. 500 mg three times a day for adults, and 250 mg for children over two to three years of age and 125 mg under this age.

The initial use of amoxycillin in children over five years of age and in teenagers is *not* ideal because the incidence of *Mycoplasma pneumoniae* pneumonia is sufficiently high in these age groups to warrant accommodation. If amoxycillin *is* used, many will of course recover (pneumococcal) but some (*M. pneumoniae*) may have a longer illness and need a subsequent antibiotic change, and a few will recover spontaneously while receiving the inappropriate antibiotic.

Augmentin

With reference to *H. influenzae*, the gain of augmentin over amoxycillin is likely to be small because the incidence of *H. influenzae* pneumonia is low; because the 6.6% incidence of ampicillin-resistant strains (Philpott-Howard and Williams 1982) although clinically significant is not high, and because only half of the resistant strains are resistant by virtue of β-lactamase production (Bell and Plowman 1980). Augmentin *is* effective against penicillin-resistant staphylococci, but whether early use in general practice would prevent illness severity in staphylococcal pneumonia is problematical. In practical terms, however, the use of augmentin for post-influenzal pneumonia is entirely acceptable.

Amoxycillin plus Flucloxacillin

An alternative option to cover the possibility of staphylococcal pneumonia while also covering *Str. pneumoniae* and *H. influenzae*, is to initially use both amoxycillin and flucloxacillin, each being given in full dosage.

Erythromycin

Erythromycin penetrates the pneumonic lung (Wollmer *et al.* 1982) and is active against *Str. pneumoniae, M. pneumoniae, Staph. aureus*, and *Legionella pneumophila. Coxiella burnetii* is resistant to erythromycin *in vitro*, but the antibiotic is effective *in vivo* (D'Angelo and Hetherington 1979, Ellis and Dunbar 1982). Conversely, *Chlamydia psittaci* is sensitive *in vitro*, but its clinical response is uncertain.

The initial use of erythromycin is the treatment of choice for children over the age of five years and for teenagers because *Str. pneumoniae* and *M. pneumoniae* are the commoner causes. The initial use of erythromycin is also a suitable alternative to amoxycillin in adults, but because *H. influenzae* is less senstive, is better confined in use to pneumonia occurring in an otherwise healthy person. Adequate dosages are 500 mg four times a day for adults and 250 mg for children over five years of age. As already argued in relation to augmentin, it is problematical whether early erythromycin use will prevent illness severity in staphylococcal pneumonia, but its use is sensible in circumstances where this type of pneumonia is possible. Similarly, the belief that erythromycin will 'cover' *Legionella pneumophila* is debatable; the severe illness requires high dose intravenous erythromycin in hospital.

Co-trimoxazole

Co-trimoxazole is active against *Str. pneumoniae* and *H. influenzae*, and its inital use is generally confined to patients who are allergic to penicillin. Whereas erythromycin is better suited to pneumonia occurring in an otherwise healthy person, co-trimoxazole is the more suitable choice for pneumonia occurring in a patient with chronic chest disease or in children under five years of age, owing to its activity against *H. influenzae*.

The Cephalosporins

Cefaclor is effective against *Str. pneumoniae, H. influenzae*, and *Staph. aureus*, but the other antibiotics already described tend to constitute an adequate therapeutic armamentarium.

Tetracycline

The initial use of tetracycline is not advised because the atypical pneumonias (*M. pneumoniae, Chlamydia psittaci*, and *Coxiella burnetii*) which do respond to tetracycline cannot be reliably diagnosed clinically; because the atypical pneumonias are uncommon (with the exception of *M. pneumoniae* in children over five years and in teenagers, as already discussed), and because *Str. pneumoniae* has an overall resistance rate of 13% to tetracycline (Ad-hoc Study Group 1977).

Conclusion

Macfarlane *et al.* (1983) have shown the value of combined intravenous ampicillin and erythromycin in hospital management and suggest that this combination is a logical initial treatment for severe pneumonia. Similarly in general practice, either amoxycillin or erythromycin are the most useful antibiotics for initial use.

Illness Course

There are three stages of recovery. Firstly the patient feels better, secondly the chest signs disappear, and thirdly the radiological evidence of pneumonia disappears. The acute stage may last three or four days and improvement is evident by loss of pyrexia, recovery of appetite, and subjectively 'feeling better'. Recovery of full health and vigour will of course take longer. Chest signs may persist for several days beyond the initial clinical recovery, and radiological evidence of pneumonia can persist for several weeks.

Antibiotic Change

The usual situation is a patient initially on amoxycillin who may now be thought to have an atypical pneumonia, and the change can be made either in the earlier stages of the illness on clinical judgement, or later when a serological diagnosis is available. Most patients do in fact recover satisfactorily, in which case the initial antibiotic is continued for a full ten days, but if the acute stage is felt to be lingering, or if slightly later in the illness chest signs are considered to be persisting, then a change may be made. The initial antibiotic must be given time to 'work', and a change is seldom made earlier than the fourth day and usually after five or six days. This is perhaps later than the timing of an antibiotic change in a severely ill patient in hospital, and reflects the less severe illness.

If the initial antibiotic was amoxycillin, the option is to change to tetracycline or erythromycin to cover the possibility of *M. pneumoniae*, psittacosis or Q-fever. In adults, tetracycline is the better choice to cover all three infective agents. In children, erythromycin will usually be chosen but it needs to be borne in mind that psittacosis might not be adequately covered. Children with an atypical pneumonia represent one of the two exceptions to the rule that tetracycline should be avoided in order to prevent staining of the secondary dentition. (The other exception is acute sinusitis - Chapter 6.)

Unresolved Pneumonia

Unresolved pneumonia may sometimes be recognized by undue persistence of chest signs, but is usually denoted later by persisting radiological evidence of infection. If an underlying cause does exist, it is likely to be bronchiectasis, chronic obstructive airways disease, carcinoma of bronchus, or secondary carcinoma, but in practice most instances of apparently unresolved pneumonia simply reflect the longish time taken for radiological clearance. The optimum time for a follow-up chest X-ray is at four to six weeks. If this X-ray is taken too early, the still present evidence of infection may cause unnecessary alarm to the patient who thought he was better, and unnecessary referral to a chest clinic.

Other Treatments

The patient requires adequate rest. Pneumonia is one of the few illnesses occurring in general practice in which old-fashioned bed rest is still advisable initially, although children are often happier downstairs on the sofa. Adequate warmth is also necessary. Pleuritic pain, cardiac failure, and associated asthma may require management, and in hospital, assisted ventilation is sometimes needed. Physiotherapy would be necessary for associated pulmonary collapse or bronchiectasis, but is otherwise unhelpful. Britton *et al.* (1985) recommend its avoidance. There are no antiviral drugs available for use at home, but a small particle aerosol of ribavirin might have a place in the treatment of viral pneumonia in hospital (Knight *et al.* 1981, McClung *et al.* 1983, Hall *et al.* 1983).

Treatment of Other Causes

Antibiotic choice in measles and pertussis pneumonia follows the guidelines already discussed because *Str. pneumoniae* and *H. influenzae* are the more common causes, but children with pertussis pneumonia will invariably be hospitalized. Other rare varieties of pneumonia are also treated in hospital. Aspiration pneumonia requires metronidazole in addition to conventional management, and Gram-negative pneumonia (excluding *H. influenzae*) is treated with intravenous aminoglycosides. Chlamydial pneumonia responds to erythromycin, and lipoid pneumonia requires discontinuation of lipoid ingestion, physiotherapy and sometimes steroids.

DIFFERENTIAL DIAGNOSIS

Over and above any underlying cause (see Unresolved pneumonia) there are two recognizable clinical situations to be distinguished from pneumonia.

'Not Pneumonia'

One out of every three patients thought clinically to have pneumonia, has no radiological evidence of pneumonia. Despite its absence, the same spectrum of age, history, chest signs, and serological findings occurs, and distinction without X-ray is not possible.

In the majority, who have a normal chest X-ray, it seems likely that acute bronchiolitis is the cause, even though this disorder has not been previously recognized as occurring often in adults and older children.

Management is the same as for pneumonia. In the minority, a few instances are explained by pulmonary collapse or cardiac failure, when the relevant X-ray change is apparent.

Predominant Pleuritic Pain

This phenomenon occurs less often than 'not pneumonia' and features pleuritic pain as the initial and predominant symptom. Most patients in addition have pyrexia, some a cough, and a few dyspnoea. The particular characteristic is the paucity of clinical and radiological findings.

Pulmonary embolism in particular needs consideration, but in general practice occurs less often under the umbrella of pneumonia than is evident in hospital; the particular clinical feature is dyspnoea out of proportion to clinical or radiological findings. Occasionally 'predominant pleuritic pain' is explained by pneumonia itself or acute bronchiolitis, but most are unexplained and acute pleurisy is inferred. This diagnosis is unsatisfactory because it is made by presumption and exclusion, but patients recover with conventional antibiotic use and fail to develop anything else. Other causes of pleuritic pain include Bornholm disease, cardiac infarction, pericarditis, spontaneous pneumothorax, herpes zoster, thoracic disc prolapse and Tietze's syndrome.

REFERENCES

Ad-hoc Study Group (1977). Tetracycline resistance in pneumococci and group A streptococci. *Br. Med. J.*, **1**, 131-133

Beem, M. O. and Saxon, E. M. (1977). Respiratory tract colonization and a distinctive pneumonia syndrome in infants infected with *Chlamydia trachomatis*. *N. Engl. J. Med.*, **296**, 306-310

Bell, S. M. and Plowman, D. (1980). Mechanisms of ampicillin resistance in *Haemophilus influenzae* from respiratory tract. *Lancet*, **1**, 279-280

Britton, S., Bejstedt, M. and Vedin, L. (1985). Chest physiotherapy in primary pneumonia. *Br. Med. J.*, **290**, 1703-1704

Communicable Disease Report (1983a). Respiratory syncytial virus infection in the elderly 1976-82. *Br. Med. J.*, **287**, 1618-1619

Communicable Disease Report (1983b). Para-influenza infections in the elderly 1976-82. *Br. Med. J.*, **287**, 1619

D'Angelo, L. J. and Hetherington, R. (1979). Q-fever treated with erythromycin. *Br. Med. J.*, **2**, 305-306

Dhillon, P. and Collins, J. (1983). Recent developments in pneumonia. *The Practitioner*, **227**, 1695-1705

Dorff, G. L., Rytel, M. W., Farmer, S. G. and Scanlon, G. (1973). Etiologies and characteristic features of pneumonias in a municipal hospital. *Am. J. Med. Sci.*, **266**, 349-358

Ellis, M. E. and Dunbar, E. M. (1982). In vivo response of acute Q-fever to erythromycin. *Thorax*, **37**, 867-868

Everett, M. T. (1983). Major chest infection managed at home. *The Practitioner*, **227**, 1743-1754

Fallon, R. J. (1983). Legionella infection in Scotland 1981-2. *Br. Med. J.*, **287**, 1469-1470

Fenton, P. A., Spencer, R. C., Savill, J. S. and Grover, S. (1983). Pneumococcal bacteraemia in mother and son. *Br. Med. J.*, **287**, 529-530

Foy, H. M., Kenny, G. E., McMahan, R., Mansey, A. M. and Grayston, J. T. (1970) *Mycoplasma pneumonoae* pneumonia in an urban area. Five years of surveillance. *J. Am. Med. Assoc.*, **214**, 1666-1672

Gratten, M., Naraqi, S. and Hansman, D. (1980). High prevalence of penicillin-insensitive pneumococci in Port Moresby, Papua New Guinea. *Lancet*, **2**, 192-195

Guarino, J. R. (1980). Auscultatory percussion of the chest. *Lancet*, **1**, 1332-1334

Hall, B. B., McBride, J. T., Walsh, E. E., Bell, D. M., Gala, C. L., Hildreth, S., Ten Eyck, L. G. and Hall, W. J. (1983). Aerolised ribavirin treatment of infants with respiratory syncytial viral infection. *N. Engl. J. Med.*, **308**, 1443-1447

Horn, M. E. C., Brain, E., Gregg, I., Yealland, S. J. and Inglis, J. M. (1975). Respiratory viral infection in childhood. A survey in general practice, Roehampton 1967-1972. *J. Hyg. Camb.*, **74**, 157-168

Isaacs, D. (1984). Psittacosis. *Br. Med. J.*, **289**, 510-511

Jacobs, M. R. and Koornhof, H. K. (1978). Multiple-antibiotic resistance - now the pneumococcus. *J. Antimicrob. Chemother.*, **4**, 481-488

Jolly, H. (1984). Tragedies in childhood. *Update*, **28**, 29-33

Knight, V., McClung, H. W., Wilson, S. Z., Waters, B. K., Quarles, J. M., Cameron, R. W., Greggs, S. E., Zerwas, J. M. and Couch, R. B. (1981). Ribavirin small-particle aerosol treatment of influenza. *Lancet*, **2**, 945-949

McClung, H. W., Knight, V., Gilbert, B. E., Wilson, S. Z., Quarles, J. M. and Divine, G. W. (1983). Ribavirin aerosol treatment of Influenza B virus infection. *J. Am. Med. Assoc.*, **249**, 2671-2674

Macfarlane, J. T., Finch, R. G., Ward, M. J. and Macrae, A. D. (1982). Hospital study of adult community acquired pneumonia. *Lancet*, **2**, 255-258

Macfarlane, J. T., Finch, R. G., Ward, M. J. and Rose, D. H. (1983). Erythromycin compared with a combination of ampicillin and amoxy-

cillin as initial therapy for adults with pneumonia including Legionnaires' disease. *J. Infect.*, **7**, 111-117
Marrie, T. J., Haldane, E. V., Noble, M. A., Faulkner, R. S., Martin, R. S. and Lee, S. H. S. (1981). Causes of atypical pneumonia: results of a 1-year prospective study. *Can. Med. Assoc. J.*, **125**, 1118-1123
Nagington, J. (1984). Psittacosis/ornithosis in Cambridgeshire 1975-1983. *J. Hyg. Camb.*, **92**, 9-19
Pether, J. V. S., Noah, N. D., Lau, Y. K., Taylor, J. A. and Bowie, J. C. (1984). An outbreak of psittacosis in a boys' boarding school. *J. Hyg. Camb.*, **92**, 337-343
Philpott-Howard, J. and Williams, J. D. (1982). Increase in antibiotic resistance in *Haemophilus influenzae* in the United Kingdom since 1977: report of a study group. *Br. Med. J.*, **284**, 1597-1599
Rachappa, B., Murthy, H. S. N. and Rogers, W. F. (1984). A case of lipoid pneumonia. *The Practitioner*, **228**, 519-522
Salmon, M. M., Howells, B., Glencross, E. J. G., Evans, A. D. and Palmer, S. R. (1982). Q-fever in an urban area. *Lancet*, **1**, 1002-1004
Schachter, J., Grossman, M., Holt, J., Sweet, R., Goodner, E. and Mills, J. (1979). Prospective study of chlamydial infection in neonates. *Lancet*, **2**, 377-379
Shann, F., Gratten, M., Germer, S., Linnemann, V., Hazlett, D. and Payne, R. (1984). Aetiology of pneumonia in Goroka Hospital, Papua New Guinea. *Lancet*, **2**, 537-541
White, R. J., Blainey, A. D., Harrison, K. J. and Clarke, S. K. R. (1981). Causes of pneumonia presenting to a district general hospital. *Thorax*, **36**, 566-570
Wollmer, P., Pride, N. B., Rhodes, C. G., Saunders, A., Pike, V. W., Palmer, A. J., Silvester, D. J. and Liss, R. H. (1982). Measurement of pulmonary erythromycin concentration in patients with lobar pneumonia by means of positron tomography. *Lancet*, **2**, 1361-1363
Yu, V. L., Kroboth, F. J., Shonnard, J., Brown, A., McDearman, S. and Magnussen, M. (1982). Legionnaires' disease: New clinical perspective from a prospective pneumonia study. *Am. J. Med.*, **73**, 357-361

11
Bronchitis, Bronchiolitis and Bronchiectasis

Acute Bronchitis - Acute Bronchiolitis - Chronic Bronchitis - Bronchiectasis

ACUTE BRONCHITIS

Acute bronchitis epitomizes the problem of trying to relate a clinical picture to a pathological term. Some doctors would apply the label to an acute respiratory viral illness without chest signs, while others would demand the presence of rhonchi or rhales, but neither interpretation is ideal because pneumonia can minic both. To add to the confusion, a flare-up of chronic bronchitis may be called acute bronchitis, and in America wheezy bronchitis is called acute bronchitis. The term is useless for both communication and antibiotic decision. The acute respiratory illnesses which may result in pathologically defined acute bronchitis are caused by a wide range of infective agents producing differing clinical pictures (Chapter 8), and patients with these illnesses can be very adequately managed without recourse to the term at all. The pesence of signs, i.e. rhonchi or rhales, would justify antibiotic use.

ACUTE BRONCHIOLITIS

Infants

Acute bronchiolitis is most commonly caused by the respiratory syncytial virus (RSV) and is the major cause of hospital admission among small children with respiratory tract infection. A preceding cold and/or cough develops after a day or two into a recognizable major chest infection with bronchospasm. Distinction from a less common pneumonia is not possible without X-ray.

Management and Antibiotic Use

Hospital admission is necessary and the ability to make a rapid viral diagnosis by immunofluorescence of naso-pharyngeal aspirate emphasizes that oxygen and supportive measures are the basis of treatment. Secondary bacterial infection is uncommon, but an antibiotic with activity against *Haemophilus influenzae* and *Streptococcus pneumoniae* (e.g. amoxycillin, cefaclor, co-trimoxazole) may be given if the distinction between bronchiolitis and pneumonia is initially uncertain. The antiviral drug ribavirin delivered as a fine particle aerosol improved the course of disease in infants with RSV pneumonia (Hall *et al.* 1983), and might also have a role in bronchiolitis.

Prevention

Risk factors include low economic status, poor housing, overcrowding, maternal smoking, other children in the family (especially an older child in the same bedroom), low birth weight and poor maternal care. As discussed in Chapter 8, p. 109, breast feeding has a smaller protective effect than believed, because the very fact that a child *is* breast fed implies a reverse of the risk factors.

Other Age Groups

Acute bronchiolitis in adults and children is likely to be more common than realized (see 'Not Pneumonia', Chapter 10). The illness both resembles and is treated as pneumonia.

CHRONIC BRONCHITIS
Clinical Features
Chronic Obstructive Airways Disease (COAD)

While predominant chronic bronchitis or predominant emphysema can occur, the two states more commonly co-exist, and it is better to think of the whole disease complex as reversible or irreversible obstructive airways disease (Nariman 1984), because this terminology is a constant reminder that there can be a reversible element. The reversible element is asthma, and the importance of remembering, recognizing, treating, and then preventing the asthma component in this illness cannot be over-emphasized.

As graphically described by Harries and Collins (1983), the patient is usually male, aged 50–60 years, who has smoked all his adult life. He has had to retire prematurely or has had to accept lighter employment. He cannot easily walk to the pub, the shops, or to the bus stop, and his wife has to do the gardening. He has increasingly frequent episodes of chest infection or cardiac failure, and to cap it all, he knows it's his own fault (i.e. smoking).

Differential Diagnosis

COAD needs to be distinguished from bronchiectasis, and it may be necessary to consider extrinsic allergic alveolitis (Chapter 10) and the industrial diseases causing progressive dyspnoea. Distinction from predominant chronic asthma may be an ideal, but is less relevant in terms of practical management because treatment is the same as for the asthma component in COAD. The rare hereditary alpha-1 antitrypsin deficiency causes severe emphysema in a younger age range of 30–40 years (McGavin 1983).

Complications

Over and above acute exacerbations of secondary bacterial infection induced by respiratory viruses, a spontaneous pneumothorax can result from rupture of an emphysematous bulla, and cardiac and respiratory failure reflect the progression of the disease or may complicate an exacerbation of infection.

Investigation

Peak flow readings serve as a base-line for subsequent bronchodilation. Chest X-ray may show an emphysematous bulla, and will help to exclude pulmonary tuberculosis and bronchial carcinoma. A blood count will demonstrate anaemia which would contribute to the dyspnoea.

Management and Antibiotic Use

Management of Asthma

Apart from advice, encouragement and sometimes insistence that smoking be discontinued, the adequate management of asthma is the single most useful thing a general practitioner can do for a patient with chronic obstructive airways disease.

Manifest Asthma

Milder degrees of illness may be controlled by regular beclomethasone and optional salbutamol, but both 'prevention' and 'treatment' are likely to be necessary, and two puffs of a β-adrenergic inhaler (e.g. salbutamol) may conveniently be followed by an adequate dose of beclomethasone, each given four times a day. Eight puffs of salbutamol per 24 hours may be safely exceeded if necessary, and 800 μg of beclomethasone by rotahaler in 24 hours is a likely minimum effective dose (400 μg twice daily might be more convenient than 200 μg four times a day). Higher doses of 1500–2000 μg (e.g. by Becloforte Inhaler) may be necessary and the small risk of adrenal suppression has to be accepted. A theophylline twice daily might be added, and the anticholinergic inhaler ipratropium bromide might be used instead of, or as well as, salbutamol.

Older people with arthritic fingers may be unable to activate an inhaler or turn a rotahaler, and because oral drugs are likely to be inadequate, the use of nebulized salbutamol at home could then be advisable, and would of course be indicated also for any patient with COAD if other methods of management were ineffective. If long-term low-dose steroids become necessary, the risk of adrenal suppression again has to be accepted, and there is need to be aware of exacerbating an existing peptic ulcer, or causing a flare-up of old tuberculosis.

Exacerbation of Asthma

Exacerbations occur in association with exacerbations of infection. Prednisolone 20 mg stat is followed by 10 mg three times daily until control is achieved (usually 48 hours) and the dose is then tailed down over the next three or four days. Alternative options include nebulized salbutamol (which might be used as well as steroids) and intravenous aminophylline, but use of the latter in a patient already taking theophylline can cause theophylline toxicity (Woodcock *et al.* 1983, Stewart *et al.* 1984).

Unrecognized Asthma

Dyspnoea at night and prolonged recovery from dyspnoea after exercise are suggestive, and as in other age groups, the physical sign of particular value is the demonstration of wheeze on forced expiration. The trial use of bronchodilators is advisable if asthma is suspect, coupled with peak flow readings. Ultimately, proof of reversibility may require a steroid trial, e.g. prednisolone 10 mg three times daily for up to two weeks. Absence of response indicates predominant emphysema and irreversibility, but the criterion is not absolute; benefit might yet be gained from nebulized salbutamol.

Antibiotic Use

Should Antibiotics be used for Acute Exacerbations?

The question may sound silly, yet the topic is controversial. A general practitioner's impression is that any of the commonly used antibiotics are effective, and this could mean that all are indeed effective or that none are. It is theoretically possible for all to be effective because most strains of *Str. pneumoniae* and *H. influenzae* will respond, but if the alternative applies, recovery is either spontaneous or achieved by other therapeutic agents. The trial by Nicotra *et al.* (1982) suggested that bronchodilators and steroids had greater relevance than antibiotics, and this implication is of interest because it echoes the management philosophy of wheezy bronchitis in children. Despite this implication, antibiotics *should* be used in the management of acute exacerbations for three reasons. Firstly, the clinical differentiation between a mild exacerbation and a more severe infection may be difficult in the presence of bronchospasm or emphysema. Secondly, the lower respiratory tract is particularly susceptible to secondary bacterial infection in COAD, the risk being greater than would occur in a child with wheezy bronchitis. Thirdly, in a patient with severe respiratory disablement, it is wrong to withhold an antibiotic on a controversial basis.

Bacteriology and Antibiotic Use

Str. pneumoniae and *H. influenzae* are the commonest pathogens. *Branhamella catarrhalis* can also become pathogenic (Slevin *et al.* 1984) in the presence of chronic chest disease, oropharyngeal aspiration, or relative immunosuppression (diabetes, rheumatoid arthritis, malignancy, alcoholism, steroid use), and because many of these organisms produce β-lactamase (Thornley *et al.* 1982, McLeod *et al.* 1983, Slevin *et al.* 1984), ampicillin and amoxycillin are inappropriate therapy. *Branhamella catarrhalis* is sensitive to erythromycin, co-trimoxazole, tetracycline and cefuroxime. Augmentin would also be effective.

Either co-trimoxazole or augmentin are the most widely suitable choices. As already argued in relation to pneumonia (Chapter 10), the gain of augmentin over amoxycillin in the treatment of *H. influenzae* is small, but because the incidence of *H. influenzae* is higher in patients with COAD, the gain is proportionately higher also. Erythomycin, tetracycline and cefaclor are active against only two of the three organisms, erythromycin being less effective against *H. influenzae*; tetracycline less active against *Str. pneumoniae*, while the effect of cefaclor on *Branhamella catarrhalis* is not clear. In the absence of *Branhamella catarrhalis*, ampicillin or amoxycillin are suitable, bearing in mind the *H. influenzae* resistance rate of 6.6%.

A remaining option is high dose amoxycillin (Cole *et al.* 1983). The authors suggest that 3 g twice daily for a short period might be more effective than conventional doses for a longer period.

Long-term Prophylaxis

The progress of the disease is not halted but there is conflicting evidence of the extent to which the number and duration of acute exacerbations are reduced (Medical Research Council 1966, Sugden *et al.* 1975). Long-term prophylaxis is best confined to those with very frequent exacerbations, with persistent purulent sputum, or if respiratory function is so reduced that further deterioration could be fatal.

Other Treatments

Oxygen needs to be given for at least 15 hours per day if survival is to be prolonged, and is therefore largely used on a short-term intermittent and symptomatic basis. There is likely to be a placebo effect. Concentrations should not exceed two litres per minute because the respiratory centre ignores the raised pCO_2 levels and is driven by hypoxaemia. Mucolytic drugs reduce the viscosity and elasticity of mucus, but do not improve lung function tests (Aylward *et al.* 1980, Tattersall *et al.* 1983), and the general feeling is that they are helpful but not of critical value. Graduated exercise induces confidence and an increased tolerance of the sensation of dyspnoea (McGavin *et al.* 1977).

BRONCHIECTASIS

Clinical Features

The characteristic feature is a chronic cough productive of copious amounts of sputum which is often purulent, and superimposed on this background, respiratory viral infections will trigger episodes of chest infection which may be recognized clinically as pneumonia. Patients with bronchiectasis are well-known in a practice, but if previously well and presenting for the first time will often present as unresolved pneumonia. Severe bronchiectasis presents problems similar to, and can also be caused by cystic fibrosis.

Management and Antibiotic Use

Postural Drainage

Postural drainage is essential and the practicality of its use can be tailored to fit the patient's needs and occupation, e.g. at home, or in a factory medical centre. Those older or more severely affected will usually attend a physiotherapy department three times a week.

Surgery

The most suitable patients for lobectomy or segmental resection are children and young adults in whom the bronchiectasis is confined to a single lobe or segment.

Antibiotic Use

The limitations of sputum culture in patients with pneumonia have already been discussed but in patients with bronchiectasis sputum culture is advisable, is likely to be helpful and is sometimes essential.

Mild Bronchiectasis

These patients will tend to have a small localized area of bronchiectasis; will have long periods of quiescence, and sputum will become purulent only during the infrequent flare-ups of infection. The bacteria isolated from the sputum during such flare-ups will usually be *Str. pneumoniae* and/or *H. influenzae*, and suitable antibiotics include amoxycillin, augmentin, co-trimoxazole and cefaclor.

More Severe Bronchiectasis

Patients more severely affected are likely to have purulent sputum all the time, and distinction between quiescence and flare-up is small. The patient will often be aware of a temporary worsening in the absence of frank pneumonia, owing to an increase in the amount of sputum or the way in which he feels. There could seem to be a role for long-term antibiotic use, but owing to the risk of inducing resistant bacterial strains, such use is confined to those with rapidly recurring flare-ups. Antibiotics are therefore given as intermittent courses, sometimes frequently. In many patients *H. influenzae* is the responsible pathogen, but other bacteria may occur, i.e. *Str. pneumoniae, Staphylococcus aureus, Pseudomonas* species and *Klebsiella* species. Although *H. influenzae* is a common cause, the commonly used antibiotics including augmentin tend to be less effective than might be expected. Doxycycline is sometimes helpful, and is likely to owe this effect to its ability to penetrate purulent material.

The sometimes limited effect of conventional antibiotics would seem to be related to dose. Cole *et al.* (1983) gave high dose amoxycillin (3 g twice daily for seven days) to 17 patients with bronchiectasis and achieved a striking clinical, spirometric, and bacterial improvement in 11 of 12 patients from whose sputum *H. influenzae* was isolated. In a subsequent study of 58 patients responding to high dose amoxycillin (representing about 60% of those treated for exacerbations over one year), Cole and Roberts (1983) found a measureable fall in the mean number and duration of exacerbations per year, and the findings of Stockley and Hill (1984) support the concept of high dose amoxycillin for those more severely ill.

Despite these findings, there is a reluctance to use high doses, generated perhaps by anticipation of side effects, but of the 17 patients treated by Cole *et al.* (1983) only one had diarrhoea and one nausea. If used within the confines of commonsense, high dose amoxycillin represents a valuable treatment method for exacerbations of infection in muco-purulent or purulent sputum producers, and is available for use in both hospital and general practice.

Cystic Fibrosis

Today many patients with cystic fibrosis survive into adolescence and adult life, and severe bronchiectasis is a common feature. The three most commonly occurring bacteria are *Staph. aureus, Pseudomonas aeruginosa* and *H. influenzae*. Children can be maintained on long-term half-dose flucloxacillin, but hospital management will usually be necessary for exacerbations and sputum culture is essential. Flucloxacillin, erythromycin, or fusidic acid are used for staphylococcal infection, while the aminoglycoside and/or carbenicillin, sometimes as a nebulized aerosol (Hodson *et al.* 1981), are used for *Ps. aeruginosa* infection.

REFERENCES

Aylward, M., Maddock, J. and Dewland, P. (1980). Clinical evaluation of acetylcysteine in the treatment of patients with chronic obstructive bronchitis: a balanced double-blind trial with placebo control. *Eur. J. Respiratory Dis.*, 61 (Suppl.) 81-89

Cole, P. J. and Roberts, D. E. (1983). High dose antibiotic is logical, effective, and economical in the treatment of severe bronchial sepsis. *Lancet*, 1, 248-249

Cole, P. J., Roberts, D. E., Davies, S. F. and Knight, R. K. (1983). A simple oral antimicrobial regimen effective in severe chronic bronchial suppuration associated with culturable *Haemophilus influenzae*. *J. Antimicrob. Chemother.*, 11, 109-113

Hall, C. B., McBride, J. T., Walsh, E. E., Bell, D. M., Gala, C. L., Hildreth, S., Ten Eyke, L. G. and Hall, W. J. (1983). Aerolised ribavirin treatment of infants with respiratory syncytial viral infection. *N. Engl. J. Med.*, 308, 1443-1447

Harries, D. and Collins, J. (1983). Rationalised treatment of COAD. *The Physician*, **1**, 364–366

Hodson, M.E., Penketh, A.R.L. and Batten, J.C. (1981). Aerosol carbenicillin and gentamicin treatemnt of *Pseudomonas aeruginosa* infection in patients with cystic fibrosis. *Lancet*, **2**, 1137–1139

McGavin, C.R., Gupta, S.P., Lloyd, E.L. and McHardy, G.J.R. (1977). Physical rehabilitation for the chronic bronchitic: results of a controlled trial of exercises in the home. *Thorax*, **32**, 307–311

McGavin, C. (1983). Chronic bronchitis and emphysema. *1983 Members' Reference Book*, The Royal College of General Practitioners. 297–299

McLeod, D.T., Ahmed, F., Power, J.T., Calder, M.A. and Seaton, A. (1983). Bronchopulmonary infection due to *Branhamella catarrhalis*. *Br. Med. J.*, **287**, 1446–1447

Medical Research Council on Trials of Chemotherapy in Early Chronic Bronchitis. (1966). *Br. Med. J.*, **1**, 1317–1322

Nariman, S. (1984). Chronic bronchitis. *Update*, **28**, 627–633

Nicotra, M.B., Rivera, M. and Awe, R.J. (1982). Antibiotic therapy of acute exacerbations of chronic bronchitis. A controlled study using tetracycline. *Ann. Intern. Med.*, **97**, 18–21

Slevin, N.J., Aitken, J. and Thornley, P.E. (1984). Clinical and microbiological features of *Branhamella catarrhalis* bronchopulmonary infections. *Lancet*, **1**, 782–783

Stewart, M.F., Barclay, J. and Warburton, R. (1984). Risk of giving intravenous aminophylline to acutely ill patients receiving maintenance treatment with theophylline. *Br. Med. J.*, **288**, 450

Stockley, R.A. and Hill, S.L. (1984). Appropriate dose antibiotics in chronic bronchial sepsis. *Lancet*, **2**, 977–978

Sugden, J.S., Launchbury, A.P. and Darke, C.S. (1975). Weekly chemoprophylaxis in chronic bronchitis. *Clinical Trials J.*, **1**, 18–23

Tattersall, A.B., Bridgman, K.M. and Huitson, A. (1983). Acetylcysteine (Fabrol) in chronic bronchitis – A study in general practice. *J. Int. Med. Res.*, **11**, 279–284

Thornley, P.E., Aitken, J., Drennan, C.J., MacVicar, J. and Slevin, N.J. (1982). *Branhamella catarrhalis* infection of the lower respiratory tract: reliable diagnosis by sputum examination. *Br. Med. J.*, **285**, 1537–1538

Woodcock, A.A., Johnson, M.A. and Geddes, D.M. (1983). Theophylline prescribing, serum concentrations, and toxicity. *Lancet*, **2**, 610–612

12
Vomiting and Diarrhoea

Non-specific Vomiting – Gastro-enteritis – Management

NON-SPECIFIC VOMITING

This is the commonest reason for vomiting in children over the age of about one year, and the underlying cause is usually a respiratory or pyrexial illness. Vomiting can thus be a feature of the whole range of illnesses discussed in previous chapters, and emphasizes yet again that any child who is unwell should be fully examined. Vomiting also commonly accompanies cough in children, representing their method of getting rid of sputum.

GASTRO-ENTERITIS

Gastro-enteritis is characterized by the triad of vomiting, diarrhoea and abdominal colic, but there is variation in presentation and illness severity. Some patients in addition have other illness features, e.g. pyrexia and respiratory symptoms, while others exhibit less than the typical triad. The age of the patient, certain clinical features, and environmental factors may combine to limit diagnostic possibilities, but stool culture is essential for an exact diagnosis.

Cause and Antibiotic Indication

Viruses

The rotavirus is the commonest viral cause and is also the commonest of all identifiable causes in children under the age of two years. Two thirds of children have a simple respiratory illness which precedes the gastro-intestinal symptoms (Lewis *et al.* 1979), and adults may vomit without diarrhoea (Hildreth *et al.* 1981). Adenoviruses and enteroviruses (Coxsackie and Echoviruses) may also cause diarrhoea as part of a more complex illness, and other viral causes include the Norwalk-like virus ('winter vomiting disease'), astrovirus, coronovirus and calicivirus.

Salmonella

Salmonella food poisoning is caused by faecal contamination of foodstuffs from a wide range of hosts including mammals, birds, amphibia and reptiles, and is a common cause of traveller's diarrhoea. In the general practice setting, the incidence is small. All ages are affected and the diarrhoea may be blood-stained.

Antibiotic Indication

With the exception of typhoid and paratyphoid, salmonella infections do not require antibiotic treatment unless the patient is severely ill or has a bacteraemic complication, e.g. osteomyelitis. Antibiotic choice is guided by the sensitivities of the patients' organism. Antibiotics are best otherwise avoided because their use may prolong the carrier state and render the organism resistant to the antibiotic used, this resistance usually being transferable (Aserkoff and Bennett 1969), and because their efficacy *in vivo* is disappointing despite *in vitro* sensitivity. Melville (1980) has demonstrated that antibiotic use is not usually necessary. The main value of a positive stool culture is awareness of the diagnosis and epidemiological control.

Campylobacter

Campylobacter jejuni (Skirrow 1977) is now the most commonly identified bacterial cause of gastro-enteritis, occurring in all age groups but predominantly in children, with an incidence of 5-15%. The infection resembles salmonella food poisoning in being a zoonosis; poultry, cattle, sheep, pigs, cats, dogs and particularly puppies with diarrhoea represent sources of human infection. The clinical picture is not reliably distinctive. The less common severe instances can resemble salmonella or shigella infection, when the diarrhoea may be bloodstained, and rarely appendicitis can be mimicked.

Antibiotic Indication

Campylobacter is eliminated by erythromycin but it is not clear whether the patient gains clinical benefit. Owing to this uncertainty and because many patients recover spontaneously, because campylobacter enteritis cannot be reliably distinguished clinically from other causes, and because erythromycin has a diarrhoea potential of its own, the antibiotic is better not used without bacteriological identification. If at this time the patient still has symptoms then it would seem reasonable to prescribe.

Shigella

Bacilliary dysentery differs from salmonella and campylobacter infection in being spread directly or indirectly by faeces from a human case or carrier. The diarrhoea typically contains blood and muco-pus.

Antibiotic Indication

There are differing views (Haltalin 1972, Keusch 1979), but most would withhold antibiotics unless the illness is severe. Inadvertent antibiotic use may have contributed to the existing high level of bacterial resistance. If the patient is treated, an absorbable antibiotic is necessary, and sensitivity testing should be undertaken despite its unreliability. Nalidixic acid has recently been used with effect (Parry 1983, Malengreau 1984). In the general practice setting, the illness may seem more severe than commonly encountered, but the type of illness severity needing antibiotic use is more likely to occur in the tropics.

Enteropathogenic *E. coli*

This organism is an infrequent cause of gastro-enteritis in children under two years of age, and is a common cause of traveller's diarrhoea.

Antibiotic Indication

Antibiotic use is justifiable in infants because recovery is faster than occurring with rehydration alone (Thorén *et al*. 1980). Choice is based upon sensitivity testing. An antibiotic may also be used when the early distinction between enteritis and septicaemia is difficult and for the attempted control of cross-infection.

Giardia

Infection by *Giardia lamblia* affects all ages but occurs most commonly in children, and is a further cause of traveller's diarrhoea. Most illnesses are short-lived, but malabsorption can be associated with a persisting diarrhoea. Cysts are identified in the stool; it may be necessary to send several specimens.

Antibiotic Indication

Treatment is indicated using metronidazole or tinizadole, and this recommendation applies also in pregnancy because an associated malabsorption may impair fetal growth. Asymptomatic cyst excretors should also be treated and, owing to difficulties in diagnosis, a suggestive clinical picture in the absence of proof justifies treatment.

Yersinia

Yersinia enterocolitica is a Gram-negative anaerobe, most prevalent in Northern Europe, and human infection is a zoonosis. The organism is present in the intestinal flora of virtually all land vertebrates (Euro Reports 1983). Children are most commonly affected. This form of gastro-enteritis is encountered in general practice but is not often seen.

Antibiotic Indication

Antibiotic use is indicated in the severe or persistent illness. The organism is resistant to the penicillins and cephalosporins (Lambert 1984), and either co-trimoxazole or tetracycline may be used.

Cryptosporidium

This protozoan parasite causes opportunist infection in those immunologically compromised, but is now recognized as also occurring in immunologically normal people (Hunt et al. 1984). The self-limiting diarrhoea of one to two weeks is most common in children and is diagnosed by finding the oocysts. There is no effective chemotherapy.

Staphylococcal Food Poisoning

After an incubation period of hours only, the patient experiences violent vomiting followed by diarrhoea, but recovery is usually complete within 24 hours. The severity of the vomiting and diarrhoea may well cause dehydration and electrolyte loss. Antibiotic use is not indicated.

Clostridium Difficile

Although better known for its causation of antibiotic-induced pseudomembranous colitis, *Clostridium difficile* can also be a cause of gastroenteritis in small children (Ellis et al. 1984). Those with symptoms and toxin in the stool need at least five days' oral vancomycin.

Traveller's Diarrhoea

Traveller's diarrhoea is not a specific disease but is caused by one or more of the many infective agents capable of causing gastro-enteritis. Many illnesses are polymicrobial (Taylor et al. 1985). Possible causative agents not already mentioned include *Aeromonas spp., Vibrio spp., Plesiomonas shigelloides* and *Blastocystis hominis*. Infection usually occurs by food-borne transmission.

Antibiotic Indication

The clinical situation commonly presented is a patient back from abroad who still has diarrhoea. Management follows the usual practice of sending a specimen of stool to the laboratory and then using antibiotics selectively. Continued pyrexia could suggest septicaemic salmonella infection. If *G. lamblia* is suspected, metronidazole might be given in the absence of an exact diagnosis.

In order to prevent infection when travelling abroad, Turner (1984) suggests the prophylactic use of Streptotriad, but many doctors would prefer to provide a non-antibiotic remedy, e.g. loperamide for use only if necessary. Attention to food hygiene is important.

Differential Diagnosis

Infants and Children

Feeding problems may result in the small frequent green stools of underfeeding or the loose frequent stools of overfeeding (usually caused by an excess of juice or water rather than milk). Surgical causes include pyloric stenosis (vomiting) in the first six weeks of life, intussusception in older infants and acute appendicitis. Diarrhoea occurring in infants should be looked upon as 'symptom query cause' (Jolly 1984) because otitis media, pneumonia, urinary infection, appendicitis, septicaemia and meningitis can all present in this way.

Non-specific abdominal pain is a common feature of many pyrexial and respiratory viral illnesses in children. The knowledge that Influenza B can cause predominant abdominal pain in children (Kerr *et al.* 1975) implies that other viruses might do the same.

Reye's syndrome although rare (Chapter 3) causes an abrupt onset of repeated vomiting in a child or teenager who has begun to get better from a respiratory viral infection or chicken pox.

Adults

Vomiting without diarrhoea can be caused by migrane, acute labyrinthitis, uraemia, and by gastro-intestinal disorders, e.g. acute duodenal ulcer, pyloric stenosis, hiatus hernia, acute cholecystitis, acute appendicitis and intestinal obstruction. Acute diarrhoea can be caused by acute diverticulitis, strangulated femoral hernia, pelvic abscess, occasionally acute appendicitis, anxiety, and a more prolonged diarrhoea by malabsorption syndromes, Crohn's disease, ulcerative colitis and aortic aneurysm. Carcinoma of the colon typically causes a variation from the normal pattern and there may be alternating diarrhoea and constipation.

The triple combination of vomiting, diarrhoea and abdominal pain (the full triad of gastro-enteritis) is possible with any of the acute surgical abdominal emergencies including general peritonitis, but the nature of the symptomatology and the clinical findings will usually enable distinction. The triple combination with shock, and perhaps blood in the stool can be caused by septicaemia and by superior mesenteric artery occlusion.

All Age Groups

Antibiotic diarrhoea is discussed in Chapter 1. Spurious diarrhoea is caused by an impacted rectum.

MANAGEMENT

An open mind is necessary in terms of differential diagnosis, and stool culture is advisable in those with diarrhoea, but the principles of management apply to both vomiting and diarrhoea and are the same irrespective of infective cause.

Fluid and Electrolyte Balance

Maintenance of fluid and electrolyte balance is essential in all age groups irrespective of drug treatment, and in many instances represents the only management necessary pending spontaneous recovery. Hyper-natraemic dehydration in infants is now uncommon because unmodified cows' milk formulae are no longer used, but can still be caused by hyper-osmolar glucose solutions, e.g. Lucozade, and by wrongly constituted replacement fluids. The increased sodium load causes irritability, twitching, increased muscle tone and/or fits.

Simple Remedies

Boiled Water

The advocacy of boiled water belongs to a bygone age, but plain water can have initial value by reducing the osmotic load in the gut (Hughes-Davies 1984).

Eliminating Solids and Diluting Milk

In the United Kingdom, a majority of children presenting with diarrhoea and/or vomiting in the general practice setting do not have a serious illness and are not in any grave danger of becoming dehydrated, and can be very adequately managed by simple home measures. Solids are eliminated, and any fluids allowed with the proviso that milk be diluted half and half with water, and that the cream is first removed. The same principle applies to adults with milder degrees of diarrhoea and/or vomiting, and to the younger child still being bottle-fed; solids are eliminated, bottle feeds are diluted by half and given more often according to need, and any clear fluids (except Lucozade) allowed *ad lib*. The same principle also applies to non-specific vomiting.

Breast Feeding

The breast fed infant presents a dilemma because the milk cannot be diluted, and opinions have been divided about the discontinuation of breast feeding. The controversy has been resolved by Khin-Maung-U *et al.* (1985) who compared oral rehydration alone with oral rehydration plus breast feeding. Those breast fed had significantly fewer stools, smaller volume stools, a significantly smaller requirement for oral rehydration and a faster recovery.

Glucose/Electrolyte Replacement Fluids

The best-known and most widely used are Diorylate or Rehidrat, which are presented as a powder needing reconstitution, and containing glucose, salt, potassium and sodium bicarbonate. In managing a small child or infant, solid food and bottled milk are discontinued, and the replacement fluid offered hourly *ad lib* aiming for about $150\,\text{ml}\,\text{kg}^{-1}\,\text{d}^{-1}$. Vomiting may be a problem, but can usually be overcome by giving small volumes frequently. As the diarrhoea subsides, the fluid is gradually withdrawn, being replaced by half-strength milk feeds and progressing then to full strength and finally to solids. In children and adults the fluid is similarly offered *ad lib*.

An alternative is a ready-to-use replacement fluid without contained bicarbonate which is equally effective (Price *et al.* 1984, Trounce and Walker-Smith 1985), and which has the advantage of obviating errors in reconstitution; parents under stress can use a smaller water volume than recommended, or reconstitute with milk, producing a fluid of higher osmolarity which might cause hypernatraemia.

Home-made replacement fluids represent a pinch of salt and a teaspoon of sugar in 250 ml water, or can be made more accurately (Glover 1984) by using one level 5 ml teaspoon of salt and eight level 5 ml teaspoons of sugar in one litre of boiled and cooled tap water.

Indications for Use

In the United Kingdom, the particular need occurs in infants. Other age groups will benefit if the degree of diarrhoea and/or vomiting is considerable.

Problems with Use

Apart from the dangers of incorrect reconstitution, there are two particular concerns. Firstly, an infant who should be admitted to hospital might continue to be managed at home. The possibility of a different diagnosis in an infant with diarrhoea needs consideration. Secondly, the replacement fluid may be given unnecessarily. Diorylate, for example, is already recognized by some parents as a necessary 'drug' for all degrees of diarrhoea and vomiting, and is probably being over-prescribed.

Anti-Diarrhoeal Drugs

Diphenoxylate and atropine (Lomotil) and loperamide (Imodium) are both effective in symptomatically reducing the frequency and severity of diarrhoea, but loperamide is the better alternative. The use of diphenoxylate and atropine in children can be dangerous and rarely fatal (Curtis and Goel 1979), and adults may infrequently feel ill for several hours. The use of loperamide in children aged between three months and three years is now known to be effective and safe in a dose of 0.4–$0.8\,mg\,kg^{-1}d^{-1}$ (Diarrhoeal Diseases Study Group UK 1984), but should not be used routinely. The belief that anti-diarrhoeal drugs encourage the proliferation of organisms by delaying the passage of stools is unsubstantiated. Kaolin is free from side effects but the benefit from its use is small.

Anti-Vomiting Drugs

Metoclopramide (Maxolon) can cause significant side effects in children (Low and Goel 1980), and adults are not free from risk. For this reason, and because non-specific vomiting seldom persists beyond 8–12 hours and the vomiting of gastro-enteritis usually subsides after the first 12–24 hours, anti-vomiting drugs have virtually no place in the management of children, and are only rarely necessary in adults. If used, a single dose is given by intra-muscular injection.

Antibiotic Use

Antibiotic indications and choices have already been discussed, and although it might be implied that antibiotics could be used quite often, the incidence of necessary prescription in the general practice setting is very small because most instances of diarrhoea have a viral cause, because spontaneous recovery is common and because severe illnesses are seldom seen.

Prevention

Breast Feeding

Breast feeding may have a smaller protective effect than believed. As already discussed in relation to respiratory illness (Chapters 8 and 11), the apparently beneficial effect of breast feeding is largely negated when allowance is made for adverse factors, i.e. low social status, over-crowding, poor maternal care and low birth weight (Taylor *et al.* 1982). As such, the fact that a child *is* breast fed implies a reverse of these factors.

Hygiene

Sanitation, purification of water, pasteurization of milk and adequate hygiene by those dealing with foods go a long way towards prevention of infection. At home, hand washing is necessary after tending relatives with diarrhoea or sick household pets, and people who handle food as an occupation must stay off work until stool culture is negative. It is customary to insist on three consecutive negative stool cultures but this rule may be less rigidly applied to Campylobacter owing to its low transmissability and inability to multiply in food at room temperatures.

Foreign Travel

In order to avoid traveller's diarrhoea and other intestinal infections, it is advisable to boil drinking water and milk, to cook food well, to peel fruits including tomatoes and to sterilize lettuce by chlorination. Watercress, shell-fish, leftovers, food on display, street vendors and fly-infested restaurants are all better avoided.

REFERENCES

Askerkoff, B. and Bennett, J. V. (1969). Effect of antibiotic therapy in acute Salmonellosis on the faecal excretion of Salmonellae. *N. Engl. J. Med.*, **281**, 636–640

Curtis, J. A. and Goel, K. M. (1979). Lomotil poisoning in children. *Arch. Dis. Child.*, **54**, 222–225

Diarrhoeal Diseases Study Group (U.K.) (1984). Loperamide in acute diarrhoea in childhood: results of a double-blind, placebo controlled multicentre clinical trial. *Br. Med. J.*, **289**, 1263–1267

Ellis, M. E., Mandal, B. K., Dunbar, E. M. and Bundell, K. R. (1984). *Clostridium difficile* and its cytotoxin in infants admitted to hospital with infectious gastroenteritis. *Br. Med. J.*, **288**, 524–526

Euro Reports (1983). Yersiniosis. Studies 60, World Health Organisation, Regional Office for Europe, Copenhagen

Glover, S. C. (1984). Rehydration for infantile diarrhoea. *Mims Magazine*, 15th October, 55–59

Haltalin, K. C., Kusmiesz, H. T., Hinton, L. V. and Nelson, J. D. (1972). Treatment of acute diarrhoea in outpatients. *Am. J. Dis. Child.*, **124**, 554–561

Hildreth, C., Thomas, M. and Ridgeway, G. L. (1981). Rotavirus infection in an obstetric unit. *Br. Med. J.*, **282**, 231

Hughes-Davies, T. H. (1984). Diarrhoea, dehydration and drugs. *Br. Med. J.*, **289**, 1542

Hunt, D. A., Shannon, R., Palmer, S. R. and Jephcott, A. E. (1984). Cryptosporidiosis in an urban community. *Br. Med. J.*, **289**, 814–816

Jolly, H. (1984). Tragedies in Childhood. *Update*, **28**, 29–33

Kerr, A. A., Downham, M. A. P. S., McQuillan, J. and Gardner, P. S. (1975). Gastric 'flu. Influenza B causing abdominal symptoms in children. *Lancet*, **1**, 291–295

Keusch, G. T. (1979). Shigella infections. *Clinics in Gastroenterology*, **8**, 645–662

Khin-Maung-U, Nyunt-Nyunt-Wai, Myo-Khin, Thane-Toe, Mu-Mu-Khin and Tin-U. (1985). Effect on clinical outcome of breast-feeding during acute diarrhoea. *Br. Med. J.*, **290**, 587–589

Lambert, H. (1984). Intestinal infections. *Med. Internat.*, **2**, 63–68

Lewis, H. M., Parry, J. V., Davies, H. A., Parry, R. P., Mott, A., Dourmashkin, R. R., Sanderson, P. J., Tyrrell, D. A. J. and Valman, H. B. (1979). A year's experience of the rotavirus syndrome and its association with respiratory illness. *Arch. Dis. Child.*, **54**, 339–346

Low, L. C. K. and Goel, K. M. (1980). Metoclopramide poisoning in children. *Arch. Dis. Child.*, **55**, 310–312

Malengreau, M. (1984). Nalidixic acid in *Shigella dysenteriae* outbreaks. *Lancet*, **2**, 172

Melville, E. M. (1980). An epidemic of gastro-enteritis in West Lothian. *J. R. Coll. Gen. Pract.*, **30**, 293–296

Parry, H. E. (1983). Nalidixic acid for Shigellosis. *Lancet*, **2**, 1206

Price, H. V., Dodge, J. A. and Thomas, M. K. (1984). Oral rehydration without added bicarbonate for childhood gastro-enteritis. *Br. Med. J.*, **289**, 532

Skirrow, M. B. (1977). Campylobacter enteritis: a "new" disease. *Br. Med. J.*, **2**, 9–11

Taylor, B., Wadsworth, J., Golding, J. and Butler, N. (1982). Breast-feeding, bronchitis, and admissions for lower respiratory illness and gastro-enteritis during the first five years. *Lancet*, **1**, 1227–1229

Taylor, D. N., Echeverria, P., Blaser, M. J., Pitarangsi, C., Blacklow, N., Cross, J. and Weniger, B. G. (1985). Polymicrobial aetiology of traveller's diarrhoea. *Lancet*, **1**, 381–383

Thorén, A., Wolde-Mariam, T., Stintzing, G., Wadström, T. and Habte, D. (1980). Antibiotics in the treatment of gastro-enteritis caused by entero-pathogenic *Escherichia coli*. *J. Infect. Dis.*, **141**, 27–31

Trounce, J. Q. and Walker-Smith, J. A. (1985). Dextrolyte in the management of children with acute gastro-enteritis. *The Practitioner*, **229**, 80–82

Turner, A. C. (1984). Are you going abroad this year? *Mims Magazine*, 15th April, 26–31

13
PUO in Children

Definition – Emergent Diagnoses – Management and Antibiotic Use

Unexplained pyrexia occurs in children of all ages but is seen most often in those between one and five years of age.

DEFINITION

A child who presents with pyrexia alone, or with pyrexia in association with vomiting and/or headache and/or abdominal pain, and in whom clinical examination is negative may be said to have PUO. This definition allows the expectation that one of a number of known diagnoses is likely to emerge and therefore allows the outcome of the illness to be foreseen. The picture commonly seen is a child who is fully conscious and not seriously ill, but hot, and knowledge of symptomatic meaning helps to make sense of the illness. 'Lying about', sleeping more than usual, and poor appetite are non-specific features of the pyrexia and have no diagnostic meaning. Similarly, vomiting, abdominal pain, and headache are commonly non-specific features of any pyrexial illness, but a persistent or severe degree of these symptoms could of course have a different significance.

A pyrexial child with cold or cough will not usually have PUO because these symptoms already indicate a respiratory viral infection, and in most children no further 'diagnosis' will emerge, but there are exceptions. Pyrexia, cold and cough represent the early stages of measles, and in two thirds of children with a rotavirus infection the diarrhoea is preceded by respiratory symptoms. Further, otitis media, sinusitis or chest infection may all develop in a pyrexial child with cold and cough, and although technically these disorders are respiratory complications, the 'diagnosis' is not complete until they have emerged. Similarly, PUO is unlikely if the child has pyrexia with diarrhoea, because this symptom will nearly always mean gastro-enteritis, but again there are exceptions. Children with appendicitis occasionally exhibit diarrhoea, and in infants and small children particularly, vomiting and diarrhoea may represent non-specific symptoms of many different infections, e.g. otitis media, pneumonia, urinary infection, appendicitis, septicaemia and meningitis.

The definition of PUO is shown to be less precise than outlined and should be broadened to include any pyrexial child in whom the diagnosis is not yet clear, or in whom it is felt that there are more illness features yet to develop.

EMERGENT DIAGNOSES

One of several possible diagnoses may emerge and the time-scale is short. The diagnosis will usually become apparent within one to four days, and although some of the emergent 'diagnoses' are nothing more than features or complications of an underlying viral infection, the emergent feature enables adequate management.

Cold and/or Cough

The development of these symptoms reflects the whole range of 'upper respiratory illness' with the potentiality for the whole range of respiratory complications, and represents the most commonly emergent 'diagnosis'.

Otitis Media

Middle ear infection has not been seen as a solitary emergent diagnosis, but does occur in association with cold or cough.

Sinusitis

Acute antral sinusitis as the emergent diagnosis is uncommon, appears as late as the fourth day of unexplained pyrexia, and may occur either as a respiratory complication or as a solitary diagnosis. A persisting unilateral conjunctivitis is suggestive, and the eventual appearance of pus in one nostril enables diagnosis.

Tonsillitis

Development of the visible tonsillar inflammation which enables the clinical diagnosis of tonsillitis may be delayed for 24 or 48 hours after the onset of the pyrexia, and rarely the delay may be longer. The bypass phenomenon (Chapter 4) can also present as PUO.

Pneumonia

Presentation as PUO is not uncommon, and the occasional absence of cough needs to be remembered. Chest signs may become evident after two to four days, but X-ray may be necessary for diagnosis. Sometimes, despite a clear chest, the diagnosis can be suggested by unilateral pain in the chest, flank, or abdomen, or by a raised respiratory rate.

Rash

The rash of measles in a non-immunized child develops on about the fourth day of the pyrexia. The pyrexia is at its highest just before the rash appears and at this stage of the illness the child is most miserable and ill. Both pyrexia and 'unwellness' persist for about 24 hours after the appearance of the rash which lasts for three or four days. The rash of rubella develops after 24 or 48 hours pyrexia, and lasts for about two days, but milder versions of the illness occur and the typical pattern may not be evident. The rash of roseolar infantum develops after the three or four day pyrexia has subsided, and can give the impression of appearing after the child has 'got better'. Many of the Echo and coxsackie viruses may cause pyrexia and rash, and these illnesses tend to lack distinctive features. The clinical distinction between enterovirus rashes, rubella, and modified measles (occurring in an immunized child) may be impossible, and the best a general practitioner can sometimes do is to suggest possibilities. Chicken pox will occasionally present as PUO, but this occurrence is more common in adults. Hand, foot and mouth disease (Coxsackie A 16, A 10, A 5) uncommonly presents as PUO. Parvovirus infection is usually without pyrexia in children.

Gastro-Enteritis

The emergence of diarrhoea will usually mean gastro-enteritis. Rotavirus infection, bacilliary dysentery and salmonella food poisoning may present with an initial unexplained pyrexia, but most children with gastro-enteritis do not have pyrexia, presenting simply with vomiting and diarrhoea, or diarrhoea alone. Emergent diarrhoea due to other causes is less common. Diarrhoea may form part of a more complex enterovirus infection, and may also occur during adenovirus infections. 'Surgical' causes are rare, but appendicitis and intussusception should not be forgotten. In infants and small children the need is always present to recognize diarrhoea as 'symptom query cause' (Jolly 1984).

Urinary Infection

Small children with urinary infections will often have no urinary symptoms and will therefore commonly present with unexplained pyrexia, but because these infections do not occur very often, this diagnosis represents only a small proportion of children presenting with PUO. Diagnosis is important because reflux in association with infection can cause renal scarring and subsequent renal failure in adult life. That this chain of events may not always apply (*Lancet* 1983) and that the renal damage may have occurred earlier, perhaps in infancy or even before birth, does not detract from diagnostic need, and if anything emphasizes the need for diagnosis at as young an age as possible. Reflux lessens after the age of five years, as the angle of obliquity by which the ureter enters the bladder increases with growth, and it is under this age that recognition is particularly important. Girls were found to be predominantly affected under two years of age (Roberts *et al.* 1983) but McKerrow *et al.* (1984) recorded an equal incidence in both sexes under two years, although girls predominated over this age. Clinically there may be nothing except an unexplained high temperature, but unilateral abdominal pain, and wetting in a child previously dry can sometimes occur.

Of all the common disorders which may emerge from a PUO presentation, urinary infection particularly cannot be diagnosed clinically, and urine culture is therefore mandatory if a diagnosis does not rapidly become apparent.

Non-Diagnosis

A high proportion, about a third of those presenting with unexplained pyrexia, recover in 24 or 48 hours without any diagnosis. These children are presumed to have had an unidentified viral infection.

Rare Diagnoses

These diagnoses *are* rare, and include brucellosis, osteitis, malaria, toxocariasis, toxoplasmosis, subacute bacterial endocarditis, apical tooth infection, subphrenic abscess, colonization of a Spitz-Holter valve, miliary tuberculosis, malignancies, and juvenile rheumatoid arthritis. On more familiar territory, a persisting pyrexia may sometimes be caused by a common infective agent producing an unusual illness. It needs to be re-emphasized that this catalogue of illness does *not* constitute the PUO commonly seen in general practice, and that the short-term but very real 'general practice PUO' is possibly less well recognized by those orientated more towards hospital.

MANAGEMENT AND ANTIBIOTIC USE

Infants with pyrexia should be admitted to hospital because septicaemia and meningitis need consideration. Older babies of a few months old may be managed at home if they are alert when properly awake, but a close watch is needed. The principle to follow in managing a child with PUO is to advise symptomatic measures until a diagnosis becomes apparent. Parents will readily accept the absence of prescription if they understand that the child is 'all right'; that one of several diagnoses may emerge, and that the doctor will check daily until the illness is resolved.

Investigation

If the diagnosis is not apparent after two or three days, then investigation should be undertaken. Urine culture and chest X-ray will demonstrate silent urinary infection or silent pneumonia respectively; a domiciliary X-ray with an immediate telephoned result is of inestimable value. A blood count may help to distinguish viral from bacterial infection, and an infectious mononucleosis screen is worth doing although glandular fever rarely presents as PUO in children. Extra blood might conveniently be taken at the same time for the first of paired sera. If the pyrexia persists and the diagnosis remains uncertain despite investigation, then the child should be admitted to hospital.

Antibiotic Avoidance Before Diagnosis

Antibiotic avoidance before diagnosis is advisable for three reasons. Firstly, several of the emergent diagnoses cannot be helped by antibiotic treatment. Secondly, urinary infection can be masked. Although the child gets better, the diagnosis is lost and with it the opportunity of perhaps identifying reflux. Inadvertent antibiotic use in this way could mean that an apparent first episode of urinary infection may in fact be the second or third episode. Thirdly, the diagnosis can be confused because emergent diarrhoea could represent either gastroenteritis or an antibiotic side effect, and an emergent rash either exanthem or allergy.

Antibiotic Use Before Diagnosis

Although antibiotic avoidance before diagnosis is preferable, exceptions do occur. An example is a child in whom acute sinusitis is going to become apparent late, and who remains hot and ill with perhaps a 'bacterial' picture in the white count. A further example would be suspected pneumonia despite a clear chest. (Immediate X-ray might not always be possible.) In such a situation it could be wrong to withhold an antibiotic from an ill child *but* in order to avoid masking a silent urinary infection, urine for bacteriology should be collected before the first dose.

Antibiotic Use After Diagnosis

The principles of management are the same whether a particular diagnosis is emergent from PUO or evident from the start of the illness. Antibiotics are used selectively as discussed in previous chapters.

Measles

Prophylactic antibiotic use is unhelpful. The child needs to be seen daily until the temperature has subsided in order to check the ears and chest. Some children may already be taking an antibiotic given in the prodromal phase for tonsillitis (see Chapter 4) or for an earlier complicating otitis media.

Urinary Infection

The child is treated according to the sensitivities of the infecting organism which is nearly always *E. coli*. Most strains are sensitive to co-trimoxazole, trimethoprim, nitrofurantoin or nalidixic acid. Beyond this, however, the aim is to prevent further episodes of infection and to consider the need for investigation to identify ureteric reflux or structural abnormality. There has long been controversy about the timing of investigation. Recommendations for IVP and micturating cystogram after a first episode (Smellie *et al*. 1964, Curran and Boston 1984, McKerrow *et al*. 1984, Jones 1984) are balanced by argument that these recommendations reflect a highly selected group of children (Houston 1984a and b), that the child suffers discomfort, and that IVP can be dangerous. (This latter point is largely discounted by Pilling 1984.)

The controversy continues, and at present a reasonable policy for the general practitioner is to refer after the first proven episode, to refer at as young an age as possible and to refer irrespective of sex. Acknowledging however that there *is* controversy, if a child is *not* referred after the first episode, then referral *should* be made after the second, and care taken to recognize it. The mother is given an MSU bottle and instructed to collect urine during any suggestive illness, and is advised that a child will not have cystitis as she would recognize it, but may start wetting though previously dry, may exhibit vague ill health, may vomit without apparent reason or may develop a high temperature.

If a significant degree of ureteric reflux is demonstrated, the child is managed by the prophylactic use of long-term half-dose antibiotic, e.g. co-trimoxazole, trimethoprim, nitrofurantoin or nalidixic acid for one or more years until possibly the age of six years. During such long-term treatment, the urine needs to be checked periodically because the advent of resistant organisms will require antibiotic change. Severe degrees of reflux are treated by oblique re-implantation of the ureters into the bladder, or more recently, by endoscopic injection of Teflon paste behind the intra-vesical ureter (O'Donnell and Puri 1984).

REFERENCES

Curran, H. J. M. and Boston, V. E. (1984). Children with vesicoureteric reflux. Presentation and investigation. *The Practitioner*, **288**, 746–747

Houston, H. L. A. (1984a). Childhood urinary tract infection. *J. R. Coll. Gen. Pract.*, **34**, 494

Houston, H. L. A. (1984b). Urinary tract infection in children. *Br. Med. J.*, **289**, 766

Jolly, H. (1984). Tragedies in childhood. *Update*, **28**, 29–33

Jones, P. F. (1984). Urinary tract infection in children. *Br. Med. J.*, **289**, 1077

Lancet (1983). Vesicoureteric reflux: more puzzles. *Lancet*, **2**, 1467–1468

McKerrow, W., Davidson-Lamb, N. and Jones, P. F. (1984). Urinary tract infection in children. *Br. Med. J.*, **289**, 299–303

O'Donnell, B. and Puri, P. (1984). Treatment of vesicoureteric reflux by endoscopic injection of Teflon. *Br. Med. J.*, **289**, 5

Pilling, D. W. (1984). Urinary tract infection in children. *Br. Med. J.*, **288**, 1159

Roberts, K. B., Charney, E., Sweren, R. J., Ahoukai, V. I., Bergman, D. A., Coulter, M. P., Fendrick, G. M., Lachman, B. S., Lawless, M. R., Pantell, R. H. and Stein, M. T. (1983). Urinary tract infection in infants with unexplained fever: a collaborative study. *J. Paediatr.*, **103**, 864–866

Smellie, J. M., Hodson, C. I., Edwards, D. *et al.* (1964). Clinical and radiological features of urinary infection in children. *Br. Med. J.*, **2**, 1222–1226.

14
Influenza and the 'Flu-like Illness

The Influenzal Illness – Viral Causes – Differential Diagnosis – Clinical Assessment of the Patient with ' 'Flu' – Management and Antibiotic Use

Influenza caused by the Influenza A and B viruses, and the similar 'flu-like illness caused by a wide range of common viruses (Poole and Tobin 1973, Everett 1977) reflect the upper end of the viral illness spectrum, and are recognizable in adults and older children. The 'flu-like illness tends to be less severe than influenza but embraces the same wide range of clinical features and can occasionally exhibit the same degree of severity.

THE INFLUENZAL ILLNESS

In order to make sense out of a plethora of symptoms and illness features, it is convenient to consider basic features, additional features, the illness course and complications.

Basic Features

There are six basic features in the full influenzal illness:

- Pyrexia
- Myalgia   } Non-respiratory
- Headache

- Cold in the nose
- Cough   } Respiratory
- Sore throat (symptom)

Pyrexia

In influenza itself, the pyrexia is high and usually lasts for three days. Occasionally the duration extends to four days, and exceptionally to five. It is important to be aware of the expected duration of pyrexia, because an extension beyond this time means either a complication, e.g. pneumonia or a different diagnosis. In the 'flu-like illness caused by non-influenzal viruses the duration of pyrexia tends to be shorter, e.g. 48 hours and less high, but may sometimes mimic the severity and duration occurring in influenza. The pyrexial phase represents the acute phase of the illness. Rigors are not uncommon and occur particularly in Influenza A infection.

Two pyrexial patterns may be seen. In one pattern the acute phase occurs at the start of the illness, all illness features presenting together, and in the other pattern the acute phase occurs in the middle of the illness, there being an initial build-up of cold and/or cough and/or sore throat (symptom). These two different patterns are unrelated to any particular viral cause, but recognition of an expected pattern is of value in management.

Myalgia and Headache

Myalgia occurs during the acute phase of the illness, and particularly affects the back, the proximal limbs and the sides of the neck.

Headache is variable in severity, and can sometimes result in a visit request for 'migraine', when an evident pyrexia will suggest the correct diagnosis. Severer degrees of headache are seen more commonly in Influenza A and enteroviral infections, and may be associated with meningism.

Cold, Cough and Sore Throat

Cold in the nose is a common feature of both influenza and the non-influenzal respiratory viral 'flu-like illness, but is occasionally absent. Severity is variable, and the cold may sometimes grumble on for a week or two.

Cough is a constant feature, being present in every instance of influenza and in almost all the 'flu-like illnesses caused by the common respiratory viruses. It can occur as part of the acute phase, but its onset is commonly delayed. The early or late onset does not reflect any particular viral cause, but knowledge of the two illness patterns, like pyrexia, is of value in management.

Sore throat is common in both influenza and the non-influenzal 'flu-like illnesses, tending to occur early and having a variable duration. The throat is nearly always non-inflamed, and the degree of non-inflamed soreness may sometimes be severe. Tonsillitis occasionally occurs.

Additional Features

Additional features are best recognized as part of the illness rather than as complications, and include vomiting, diarrhoea, laryngitis, tracheitis, tonsillitis, chest pain, meningism and urinary symptoms. Vomiting is much less common in adults than in children, and may be associated with severe headache or meningism. Both diarrhoea and myalgic chest pain occur infrequently and tend to be associated with an enteroviral cause, but diarrhoea can be a feature of other common viral causes. Urinary frequency without discomfort is a common accompaniment of an influenzal illness and has no significance.

Tonsillitis

The sore throat of an influenzal illness will occasionally be caused by tonsillitis, which occurs particularly in adenoviral, enteroviral and herpes simplex infections. Curiously, tonsillitis is virtually absent in association with Influenza A infection.

Meningism

The phenomenon most often seen is pain in the low back induced by neck flexion, without any other meningeal feature. This finding is interpreted as very mild meningism or a 'meningeal flavour'. Meningism itself (headache, photophobia, neck stiffness) is not very common, and occurs particularly in Influenza A and enteroviral infections. Most occurrences are short-lived, but persistence over 48 hours implies viral meningitis.

Illness Course

The acute phase is represented by the pyrexia and myalgia particularly, and the duration of this phase reflects the duration of the pyrexia. The subsequent recovery phase is characterized by the continuing cough which may last for two weeks and a gradual return of energy which can take a similar length of time.

Complications

Respiratory

Respiratory complications are the most common and include chest infection, sinusitis and otitis media, all of which may be seen in both influenza and in the non-influenzal 'flu-like illness. Otitis media will tend to be present during the acute phase of the illness, but is rare in adults. Sinusitis is occasionally seen, and usually occurs later during the recovery phase in association with a lingering cold. The complication of particular relevance is pneumonia, which is heralded by persistence of pyrexia beyond the expected time, or by recrudescence of pyrexia after initial subsidence. Occasionally chest signs will be evident earlier, during the acute phase. Chest infection of lesser severity can also occur, and asthma will become more marked in those with chronic obstructive airways disease.

Cardiac

Acute myocarditis is very rare and is suggested by post-influenzal tachycardia or arrhythmias or cardiac failure. Pericarditis rarely occurs.

Post-Viral Neurological Syndromes

A brief phase of depression after ''flu' is not uncommon, but the Guillain–Barré syndrome affecting peripheral nerve myelin, and acute disseminated encephalomyelitis affecting central nervous tissue myelin (Behan 1983) are rarely seen. Possibly less rare is the post-viral fatigue state myalgic encephalomyelitis, which can probably follow several types of viral infection, and has been described in both epidemic and sporadic form following Group B coxsackie virus infection (Fegan *et al*. 1983, Keighley and Bell 1983). The extreme exhaustion, the prolonged convalescence, and the multiple symptoms including anxiety and depression may cause sufferers to be labelled neurotics.

VIRAL CAUSES
Influenza A and B

Influenza cannot be reliably distinguished from other viral causes without laboratory identification but is suggested by a rapid increase in the incidence of ''flu' during a winter or spring month. During an epidemic it is common to find more than one member of a family simultaneously affected, and to see patients who are rarely seen or have never been seen before. Clinical distinction between Influenza A and B is not possible, and the belief that Influenza B causes a milder disease is quite unfounded; this variety of influenza can be every bit as severe as Influenza A infection and can be similarly complicated by pneumonia. In outbreaks or epidemics of influenza, Influenza A and B commonly co-exist. This occurrence has relevance to studies of vaccination efficacy, and to the use of amantadine which is active only against Influenza A. During an influenza epidemic, most patients with ''flu' will indeed have influenza, but other common viruses may be present in the community at the same time (see Chapter 8, Persistent Cough) and an occasional patient may have a different diagnosis altogether.

Other Common Viruses

Rhinoviruses, adenoviruses and herpes simplex may cause a 'flu-like illness at any time of the year, whereas the respiratory syncytial virus usually appears during the winter and early spring. Enterovirus 'flu is seen mainly in the summer and autumn. Illnesses caused by parainfluenza viruses may occur at any time of the year but outbreaks tend to have summer peaks. The respiratory syncytial virus is best known for its causation of bronchiolitis in infants, but can also cause a 'flu-like illness in adults. Similarly, herpes simplex is best known for recrudescence of latent infection, but in causing a 'flu-like illness is likely to be acting as a primary invader because such patients rarely have cold sores, and paired sera demonstrate a four-fold or greater rise in titre.

Enteroviruses

Coxsackie and Echo viruses differ from other viral agents in sometimes causing a non-respiratory 'flu-like illness characterized by the triad of pyrexia, myalgia and headache. Cold and cough are absent, but about half have the symptom sore throat. Tonsillitis can occur, but in most the throat is non-inflamed. Patients with enterovirus 'flu tend to have a higher incidence of severe headache, meningism, myalgic chest pain and diarrhoea.

DIFFERENTIAL DIAGNOSIS

Most patients with ''flu' will have either influenza or a common viral cause, but there are many other disorders which may present as or be interpreted initially as ''flu'. Most are encountered only rarely. In the adult, the 'flu-like illness and PUO can merge imperceptibly. Many of the differential diagnoses are without cough. Although an absent cough can occur in enterovirus 'flu and may also reflect the delayed onset occurring in influenza itself, its absence should alert the doctor to the possibility of a different diagnosis.

Miscellaneous

Bacterial

Pneumonia from any cause, bacilliary dysentery, urinary infection, septicaemia, and acute bacterial endocarditis can all be initially interpreted as ''flu'. Acute bacterial endocarditis (Welsby 1977) is recognized in elderly patients who have aortic valve involvement of a degenerative rather than rheumatic nature.

Viral

Glandular Fever

Less common presentations among adults include PUO and an influenzal illness. This latter can embrace all six basic features including cold and cough, and unless investigation happens to be undertaken can pass unrecognized as ''flu'.

Cytomegalovirus Infection

Acquired cytomegalovirus infection occurs in teenagers and younger adults and may present with a prolonged influenza-like illness lasting two weeks or more (Nye 1984). Infection during pregnancy can cause damage to the fetal nervous system resulting in mental retardation.

Mycoplasma Pneumoniae

Mycoplasma pneumoniae infrequently causes a 'flu-like illness without chest infection in adults. The full influenzal illness can be mimicked, and unless investigated represents a second illness (ref. glandular fever) which can pass undiagnosed as ' 'flu'.

Carbon Monoxide Poisoning

The British Gas Corporation has recently (1984) reminded the medical profession that carbon monoxide poisoning still exists and can be mistaken for influenza. The cause is poor combustion compounded by inadequate flueing and ventilation, and the risk is greatest during the winter in those who are housebound.

Related to Foreign Travel

Poliomyelitis

Sporadic cases of poliomyelitis occur in the United Kingdom, but because the disease is still prevalent in tropical and sub-tropical areas particularly, it is usually contracted abroad. The milder illnesses exhibit a self-limiting 'flu-like illness without meningitis.

Malaria

70% of all malaria occurs in India and 25% in Africa, and most of the latter is caused by *Plasmodium falciparum* which can kill if not recognized and treated. About 2000 people per year develop malaria in the UK, and in about a quarter *P. falciparum* is responsible (Helliwell and Turner 1980). The patient will typically exhibit pyrexia, headache, vomiting, joint pains and a periodic fever. In recent years several patients have died, and the chain of events has invariably been a return from abroad and the development of an illness which was diagnosed as influenza. The two particular points which help to make the diagnosis are the very fact of having been abroad and an acute illness phase which persists beyond the expected time of three days. The diagnosis can be confirmed by thick and thin blood films, but if there is uncertainty in diagnosis, treatment should be given on suspicion. 'Airport malaria' (Smeaton *et al.* 1984) occurs in people who have not visited a malaria area, but have been bitten by a commuter mosquito picked up on a previous flight elsewhere.

Typhoid

About 200 people with typhoid are seen annually in the UK and nearly all the illnesses are related to foreign travel. It is in the earlier stage only that the illness could resemble or be mistaken for ' 'flu'. The continued illness beyond three or four days would soon make it evident that the patient had another diagnosis.

Legionnaires' Disease

Legionella pneumophila is similar to *M. pneumoniae* in causing either pneumonia or a 'flu-like illness, but the latter is uncommon. Legionnaires' disease can be contracted in the UK, but a third are associated with foreign travel (Chapter 10, p. 144).

Lassa Fever

Lassa fever occurs in the rural areas of Nigeria, Liberia and Sierra Leone (Helliwell and Turner 1980) and causes fever, malaise, intense toxicity and usually an exudative pharyngitis, with a degree of prostration far greater than expected.

Related to Occupation and/or Contact with Animal or Bird

Psittacosis

The infective agent, *Chlamydia psittaci*, is in keeping with *M. pneumoniae* and *Legionella pneumophila* in that it also produces either pneumonia or a 'flu-like illness without chest infection. Both types of illness occur with equal frequency. Psittacosis is a third disorder (ref. glandular fever and *M. pneumoniae*) which can pass undiagnosed as ''flu'. As discussed in Chapter 10, p. 145, birds are a source of infection, and relevant occupations include farming, veterinary work, pet shops, fish handling (gulls), and the chicken, turkey, and duck processing plants, but there is evidence also for a non-psittacine association and human to human spread.

Psittacosis from Sheep

Chlamydia psittaci is the major cause of abortion in sheep in the United Kingdom (Johnson 1983). Human infection is rare but can be contracted by the pregnant wives of sheep farmers. The organism has a prediliction for the placenta, and the septicaemic illness with intravascular coagulation can cause both maternal and fetal death (Beer *et al.* 1982). Antibiotics are ineffective, and the over-riding need is to rid the patient of the placenta, irrespective of gestational age.

Q-Fever

Coxiella burnetii is the fourth infective agent which may cause either pneumonia or a 'flu-like illness without chest infection, and is yet another infection which can pass undiagnosed as ' 'flu'. As discussed in Chapter 10, p. 146, cattle and sheep represent the reservoir of infection in Britain, and relevant occupations embrace farms, slaughter houses, hides, fleeces, and veterinary work. The disease can also be contracted abroad.

Leptospirosis

It is common for leptospirosis to present as a 'flu-like illness, and meningism may be associated. Weil's disease (*L. icterohaemorrhagiae*) occurs traditionally in sewerage workers, but may be caught by any individual contacting stagnant water in rat-infested districts, and includes bathers, canoeists, and raft racers in canals and rivers. Infected urine from pigs and dogs may also cause human infection, and the cow (*L. hebdomadis*) is now recognized as a source of infection. Wilson and Wetson (1981) describe three cases of human leptospirosis on a small dairy farm. One patients was infected by *L. icterohaemorr-*

hagiae believed caused by contact with hay contaminated by rat urine. The other two were infected by *L. hebdomadis*, and it seemed very probable that the source of their infection was cow's urine.

Brucellosis

Brucellosis is now rare in Britain because 99% of dairy herds in England, Scotland and Wales were accredited brucellosis-free in 1981 (Public Health Laboratory Service Report 1984). Herds with still active *Brucella abortus* infection were situated mainly in north-east England, Devon, Cornwall and Wales. The disease may also be contracted abroad. *B. melitensis* in goats or sheep causes infection in man by the ingestion of raw milk or milk products but *B. abortus* in cattle (*The Lancet* 1983) is more likely to be transmitted by aerosol spread from heavily contaminated material, and to enter via the respiratory tract. There is great variation in clinical presentation, but it would quickly become apparent that undulent fever was something different from influenza.

Streptococcus Suis Type II Infection

Occurring among workers in the pig industry (Clements *et al.* 1982), the clinical features are meningitis and septicaemia with sometimes purulent arthritis, and the initial presentation may reflect a 'flu-like illness.

Toxoplasmosis

Humans acquire toxoplasmosis by eating raw or undercooked meat containing the parasite in the form of inactive tissue cysts, or by ingesting mature oocytes derived from cat faeces usually via contaminated soil (Nye 1984). The commonest manifest illness is characterized by painless enlargement of lymph nodes, particularly in the neck, but presentation as a 'flu-like illness can occur, sometimes with meningism. The particular concern is the fetus. Just as farmers' wives who are pregnant should not help with lambing in order to avoid catching psittacosis from sheep, so also should pregnant women avoid contact with cats and avoid eating raw or partly cooked meats in order to prevent congenital toxoplasmosis.

Extrinsic Allergic Alveolitis

The granulomatous inflammation of respiratory bronchioles and alveoli progresses eventually, if unchecked, to pulmonary fibrosis. The cause is a local allergic reaction to inhaled organic dusts, particularly fungal spores and animal protein (Davison and Newman Taylor 1983), and embraces farmer's lung, bird fancier's lung, maltworker's lung, baggassosis and mushroom worker's lung. It is the acute illness following heavy exposure which may resemble ''flu'. The dyspnoea without wheeze, fever and 'flu-like symptoms appear 4–8 hours after exposure, and on examination there are loud crackles and squeals in the chest.

PUO

If the 'flu-like illness remains unexplained or verges towards PUO, it may be necessary to think more widely in terms of malignancies, connective tissue disease, gramulomatous lesions, drug fevers, factitious illness or the more exotic tropical illnesses.

Resumé

Some of the various points made in this section are summarized in the following tables:

---

1. The pyrexia persists beyond the expected three or four days
2. The patient is more ill than expected
3. Unexpected illness features develop
4. Absent cough
5. Recent return from abroad
6. Occupation or contact with relevant animal or bird

Table 14.1 Clinical factors which may suggest a differential diagnosis in a patient with an influenzal illness

CLINICAL ASSESSMENT OF THE PATIENT WITH ''FLU'

It follows that assessment should be broad-based.

Enquiry and examination should embrace all systems, and it is

Poliomyelitis Malaria Typhoid Lassa fever	Invariably contracted abroad
Legionnaires' Disease Leptospirosis Q-fever Toxoplasmosis Brucellosis	Contracted both abroad and in the U.K.

Table 14.2 Illnesses contracted abroad which may present as ''flu'

Q-fever
Leptospirosis
Streptococcus suis type II infection
Brucellosis
Extrinsic allergic alveolitis (hay)
Psittacosis in pregnancy (sheep)

Table 14.3 Illnesses related to farming and allied occupations which may present as ''flu'

Glandular fever
Mycoplasma pneumoniae infection
Psittacosis
Q-fever
Leptospirosis

Poliomyelitis ⎱ Probably
Toxoplasmosis ⎰

Table 14.4 Illnesses which may sometimes pass undiagnosed as ''flu' unless investigation happens to be undertaken

helpful to run through in one's mind the six basic features and the possible additional features. Enquiry should be made of recent travel abroad, of occupation if this is not already known, and of contact with animals or birds whether as pets, in zoos or on farms. It takes only a moment or two to ask these questions and the problem perhaps is not in the asking but in remembering to do so. It is no longer a surprise to find

Mycoplasma pneumoniae
Legionella pneumophila
Chlamydia psittaci (Psittacosis)
Coxiella burnetii (Q-fever)

Table 14.5 Infective agents which can cause either an influenzal illness or pneumonia

that an unassuming suburban housewife has just returned from Africa. If a patient presents late, retrospective questioning will establish the duration of pyrexia.

MANAGEMENT AND ANTIBIOTIC USE

Most patients have an uncomplicated illness and can be managed symptomatically. As also in simple respiratory illness, the doctor should not be afraid to say that there is no specific treatment and that the illness has to run its course. Treatment of associated asthma may sometimes be necessary, but cough medicines are of limited value. The use of steam (Chapters 7 and 8) for an irritating cough can help adults and older children just as much as those younger. The extent of follow-up is dependent upon illness severity and clinical judgement, but the patient should certainly be seen again if the pyrexia persists beyond three days, in order to consider either complication or different diagnosis.

Meningism in an adult with an influenzal illness will invariably be viral (usually Influenza A or an enterovirus) and the need to recognize bacterial meningitis has less relevance than in children, but there is need to remember the rare differential diagnoses (poliomyelitis, Q-fever, leptospirosis, toxoplasmosis, *Str. suis* Type II infection). Home management is usually acceptable, but admission is advisable in the severe instance both for diagnosis, and because management of the prolonged headache and convalescence which follows viral meningitis is made easier if the patient has already had the reassurance of the hospital second opinion.

Investigation

Of necessity, most patients with ''flu' have no investigations and recover satisfactorily, but investigation is advisable in those with relevant animal or bird contact, with relevant occupation, in those recently returned from abroad, and if the pyrexia persists and verges on PUO. A more comprehensive identification of cause, including those which pass undiagnosed as ' 'flu', entails investigation of consecutive illnesses. The basic investigations include blood count, glandular fever sceeen test, chest X-ray, MSU, viral throat swab, paired sera, and sometimes viral and bacterial culture of stool. Blood culture is occasionally undertaken from home.

Antibiotic Use

The view which says that ' 'flu' is a viral infection and does not require antibiotic treatment is as extreme as the view which gives ampicillin to all cases without thinking. Influenza and the common viral 'flu-like illness represent the ultimate in selective antibiotic use because so many illness features may be associated. A majority of patients will *not* require antibiotics because pyrexia *per se*, headache, myalgia and cold-in-the-nose cannot be helped by antibiotic treatment, and early routine antibiotic use neither alters the course of the illness nor prevents pneumonia. Further, antibiotic treatment is rarely necessary for the non-inflamed sore throat and seldom helps the cough without chest infection. Selective antibiotic use means that a few patients will require antibiotics for associated tonsillitis; for complicating chest infection, sinusitis or otitis media, and possibly for laryngitis and painful tracheitis. A 'bad' or 'chesty' cough might also sometimes be felt to justify antibiotic use, despite a clear chest.

Just as in small children with a simple respiratory illness, knowledge of illness patterns enhances sensible prescribing. A patient with a delayed pyrexia pattern will probably cope with the initial cold, cough etc., and present when the temperature appears. If clinical examination is negative and a complication judged to be absent, then antibiotics may be withheld because the advent of pyrexia represents a normal illness pattern. Similarly, the advent of a delayed cough does not necessarily mean 'it's gone down onto my chest' but may reflect a known pattern of illness.

Antiviral Drugs

Amantadine

Amantadine is active against Influenza A, and has a role in prevention

(Dolin et al. 1982, Rose 1983, Payler and Purdham 1984), in modifying the established disease, and in preventing spread (Van Voris et al. 1981), but in order to avoid side effects the dose should be limited to 100 mg daily in both children over 10 years and in adults.

Amantadine is effective only against Influenza A, and in combined outbreaks of Influenza A and B therefore, some patients would receive the drug unnecessarily. Rapid diagnosis by immunofluorescence of naso-pharyngeal aspirate would be neither practicable nor acceptable by all patients. A further problem in an open population relates to prevention; who should receive the drug? Finally there is lack of knowledge relating to teratogenic side effects, and use in females needs to be selective. In practice, amantadine would be largely used blind, and is likely to be confined in use for closed communities or for patients particularly at risk, and as such would have indications for use similar to those currently recommended for influenza vaccination.

Ribavirin

Ribavirin delivered through a mask as a small particle aerosol improved the course of influenza in adults with established Influenza A (Knight et al. 1981) and Influenza B infection (McClung et al. 1983). Ribavirin is possibly more effective than amantadine and has the advantage that differentiation between Influenza A and Influenza B is not necessary, but the generator needed to produce the small particle size confines its use to hospital. This degree of therapeutic sophistication is quite unjustified for the 'ordinary case of influenza', but could be justified in viral pneumonia.

REFERENCES

Beer, R. J. S., Bradford, W. P. and Hart, R. J. C. (1982). Pregnancy complicated by psittacosis acquired from sheep. *Br. Med. J.*, **284**, 1156-1157

Behan, P. O. (1983). Postviral neurological syndromes. *Br. Med. J.*, **287**, 853-854

Clements, M. R., Hamilton, D. V., Clifton-Hadley, F. A. and O'Reilly, J. F. (1982). *Streptococcus suis* type II infection. A new industrial disease? *The Practitioner*, **226**, 323-325

Davison, A. G. and Newman Taylor, A. (1983). Allergies that are related to jobs. *Mims Magazine*, 15 September, 28-35

Dolin, R., Reichman, R. C., Madore, H. P., Maynard, R., Lindon, P. N. and Webber-Jones, J. (1982). A controlled trial of amantadine and rimantadine in the prophylaxis of Influenza A infection. *N. Engl. J. Med.*, **307**, 580-584

Everett, M. T. (1977). The 'flu-like illness. *The Practitioner*, **219**, 699-711

Fegan, K. G., Behan, P. O. and Bell, E. J. (1983). Myalgic encephalomyelitis - report of an epidemic. *J. R. Coll. General Practitioners*, **33**, 335-337

Helliwell, C. J. V. and Turner, A. C. (1980). Imported disease at point of entry. *The Practitioner*, **224**, 793-796

Johnson, F. W. A. (1983). Chlamydiosis. *Br. Vet. J.*, **139**, 93-101

Keighley, B. D. and Bell, E. J. (1983). Sporadic myalgic encephalomyelitis in a rural practice. *J. R. Coll. Gen. Pract.*, **33**, 339-341

Knight, V., McClung, H. W., Silson, S. Z., Waters, B. K., Quarles, J. M., Cameron, R. W., Greggs, S. E., Zerwas, J. M. and Couch, R. B. (1981). Ribavirin small-particle aerosol treatment of influenza. *Lancet*, **2**, 945-949

Lancet (1983). How does *Brucella abortus* infect human beings? *Lancet*, **2**, 1180

McClung, H. W., Knight, V., Gilbert, B. E., Wilson, S. Z., Quarles, J. M. and Divine, G. W. (1983). Ribavirin aerosol treatment of Influenza B virus infection. *J. Am. Med. Assoc.*, **249**, 2671-2674

Nye, F. (1984). The mononucleoses. *Med. Internat.*, **2**, 29-34

Payler, D. K. and Purdham, P. A. (1984). Influenza A prophylaxis with amantadine in a boarding school. *Lancet*, **1**, 502-504

Poole, P. M. and Tobin, J. O'H. (1973). Viral and epidemiological findings in MRC/PHLS surveys of respiratory disease in hospital and general practice. *Postgrad. Med. J.*, **49**, 778-787

Public Health Laboratory Service Report (1984). Brucellosis in Britain. *Br. Med. J.*, **289**, 817

Rose, H. J. (1983). Use of amantadine in influenza: a second report. *J. R. Coll. Gen. Pract.*, **33**, 651-653

Smeaton, M. J., Slater, P. J. and Robson, P. (1984). Malaria from a "commuter" mosquito. *Lancet*, **1**, 845-846

Van Vorris, L. P., Betts, R. F., Hayden, F. G., Christmas, W. A. and Douglas, R. G. Jr. (1981). Successful treatment of naturally occurring Influenza A/USSR/77 H1N1. *J. Am. Med. Assoc.*, **245**, 1128-1131

Welsby, P. D. (1977). Infective endocarditis - a retrospective study. *The Practitioner*, **218**, 382-387

Wilson, D. and Wetson, R. (1981). Leptospirosis - a diagnostic problem and an industrial hazard. *J. R. Coll. Gen. Pract.*, **31**, 165-167

Index

abdominal pain, non-specific 100, 174
absorption of antibiotics 17
adenoidal hyperplasia 72, 78, 106
adenoviruses 51, 66, 91, 100, 122, 147, 170, 193
alcoholism
  metronidazole 16
allergy
  erythromycin 5
  penicillins 1
  sulphonamides 5
  tetracycline 5
amantadine 202
aminoglycosides 14, 15, 16, 154, 167
amoxycillin
  allergy 1
  breast feeding 12
  bronchiectasis 166
  chronic obstructive airways disease 163
  contraceptive pill 7
  cough 101
  croup and laryngitis 94, 96
  high dose
    bronchiectasis 166
    chronic obstructive airways disease 164
    otitis media 76
  otitis media 75
  pneumonia 150
  pregnancy 9
  tonsillitis 58
  wheezy bronchitis 127
ampicillin
  absorption 17

allergy 1, 2
breast feeding 12
chronic obstructive airways disease 163
contraceptive pill 7
cough 101
croup and laryngitis 94, 96
pneumonia 150
pregnancy 9
sinusitis 88
tonsillitis 58
anaerobic bacteria 58, 71, 79, 87, 148
anaphylactic shock 1, 4
antiviral agents 108, 127, 154, 160, 203
aspirin 37
asthma (including wheezy bronchitis)
  aminophylline, intravenous 124, 163
  antibiotic use 126
  bronchodilators 123, 128
  chronic obstructive airways disease 160
  differential diagnosis 96, 105, 131
  deaths 126
  erythromycin and theophylline toxicity 15
  flu-like illness 192
  infants 124
  prevention 128
  recognition 122
  steroids 123, 129
  theophylline and erythromycin toxicty 15
  unrecognised 112, 115, 163
  wheezy bronchitis nature 121

augmentin
  allergy 1
  breast feeding 12
  bronchiectasis 166
  chronic obstructive airways
     disease 163
  contraceptive pill 7
  croup and laryngitis 94, 96
  otitis media 75
  pneumonia 150
  pregnancy 9
  sinusitis 88
auroscope use 65

bacterial endocarditis, acute 194
β-haemolytic streptococcus 51, 71, 79, 148
Branhamella catarrhalis 164
breast feeding
  antibiotic use when 12
  gastro-enteritis 176
  prevention, gastro-enteritis 178
  prevention, respiratory illness 109, 160
bronchiectasis 165
  antibiotic use 166
  cystic fibrosis 167
  unresolved pneumonia 153
bronchiolitis
  infants 159
  adults and children 160
bronchitis
  acute 159
  chronic (see chronic obstructive
    airways disease)
brucellosis 198

campylobacter 170
candida 49
carbenicillin 167
carbon monoxide poisoning 195
carcinoma of bronchus 115, 153, 161
cardiac failure 137, 154
central heating 114
cephalosporins
  allergy
    cross reaction in penicillin
      allergy 3
  breast feeding 12
  cefaclor
    bronchiectasis 166
    chronic obstructive airways
      disease 164

croup 94
otitis media 76
pneumonia 152
sinusitis 88
contraceptive pill 7
elderly 14
neonates 13
pregnancy 9
tonsillitis 57
chicken pox 148, 183
children
  teeth staining by tetracycline 13
Chlamydia psittaci
  flu-like illness 196
  pneumonia 145
  psittacosis from sheep 197
Chlamydia trachomatis 72, 149
chloramphenicol
  croup 94
  warfarin 16
chlorpropamide
  antibiotic toxicity 16
chronic obstructive airways disease 160
  antibiotic use 163
  asthma 161, 162, 192
  bacteria 164
  unresolved pneumonia 153
cold in the nose 105
  antibiotic use 107
  differential diagnosis 106
  flu-like illness 190
  infants 108
  PUO 182
contraceptive pill
  antibiotic interaction
    combined pill
    progesterone only pill 8
cot death 36, 38, 108
co-trimoxazole
  absorption 17
  allergy 5
  breast feeding 12
  bronchiectasis 166
  chronic obstructive airways
    disease 163
  contraceptive pill 7, 8
  cough 101
  croup 94
  diabetes 16
  elderly 14
  methotrexate 16
  neonates 13
  otitis media 76

Index

pneumonia 151
pregnancy 10
sinusitis 88
tonsillitis 57
urinary infection 187
warfarin 16
wheezy bronchitis 126
yersinia 172

cough
  absent 116, 137, 194
  acute 100
  allergic 113
  asthma (unrecognised) 112, 115
  bronchiectasis 165
  bronchiolitis 159
  bronchitis 159, 160
  carcinoma of bronchus 115
  central heating 114
  cystic fibrosis 114
  flu-like illness 190
  gas cooking 114
  hiatus hernia 116
  inhaled foreign body 105
  measles 103
  Mycoplasma pneumoniae 104
  persistent in adults 114
  persistent in children 109
  pertussis 103, 110, 116
    antibiotic uses 104, 110
  pneumonia 135
  PUO 182
  rare causes 114
  recurrent 109, 113
  rotavirus 103
  smoking, passive 114
  tuberculosis 115
Coxiella burnetii
  flu-like illness 197
  pneumonia 146
coxsackie viruses 51, 100, 106, 121, 170, 183, 193
croup (see laryngitis)
cryptosporidium 173
cystic fibrosis 114, 167
cytomegalovirus 194

delirium 34
diabetes 16
diagnostic labels 21
diarrhoea
  antibiotic induced 5
    pseudomembranous colitis 6

gastro-enteritis 169
  antibiotic use 169, 178
  antidiarrhoeal drugs 177
  breast feeding 176, 178
  campylobacter 170
  Clostridium difficile 173
  cryptosporidium 173
  enteropathogenic *E. coli* 171
  fluid balance 175
  Giardia lamblia 172
  PUO 184
  salmonella 170
  shigella 171, 194
  Staphylococcus aureus 173
  traveller's diarrhoea 173
  viruses 169
  yersinia 172
  symptom of another cause 174
digoxin
  antibiotic toxicity 14
diphtheria 49
doxycycline
  breast feeding 12
  bronchiectasis 166
  contraceptive pill 7
  elderly 14
  epilepsy 16
  pregnancy 11
  sinusitis 88
  teeth staining 13

earache
  differential diagnosis 70
echoviruses 51, 100, 106, 121, 170, 183, 193
elderly
  antibiotic use when 14
emphysema (see chronic obstructive airways disease)
encephalomyelitis, acute disseminated 192
epilepsy
  doxycycline 16
epiglottitis 92
erythromycin
  allergy 5
  breast feeding 12
  campylobacter 170
  chronic obstructive airways disease 163
  cystic fibrosis 167
  jaundice risk 10
  otitis media 74

erythromycin *cont.*
  pertussis 103, 110
  pneumonia 151, 152
  pregnancy 10
  sinusitis 88
  theophylline toxicity 15
  tonsillitis 57
  wheezy bronchitis 126
extrinsic allergic alveolitis 161, 199

febrile convulsions 31
fever (see pyrexia)
flucloxacillin
  cystic fibrosis 167
  neonates 13
  pneumonia 151
flu-like illness 189
  antibiotic use 202
  antiviral agents 202
  clinical assessment 199
  complications 192
  differential diagnosis 194
  investigation 201
  meningism 191, 201
  viruses 193
folic acid deficiency 10
fusidic acid 167

gas cooking 114
gastro-enteritis (see diarrhoea)
Giardia lamblia 172
glandular fever 48, 58, 194
glucose-6-phosphate dehydrogenase deficiency 11, 12
Gram negative bacteria (excluding *H. influenzae*) 79, 148, 166, 167, 171, 187
Guillain-Barré syndrome 192

Haemophilus influenzae 71, 79, 86, 92, 106, 147, 164, 166, 167
Haemostasis
  antibiotic influence 16
hand, foot and mouth disease 183
hepatic failure and antibiotics 15
  breast feeding 13
  erythromycin jaundice 10
  tetracycline and chlorpropamide 15
herpes simplex 51, 66, 100, 193
hiatus hernia 116

immunosuppression 72, 149, 164

infectious mononucleosis (see glandular fever)
influenza (see flu-like illness)
influenza viruses 51, 66, 91, 100, 121, 147, 193
inhaled foreign body 105

jaundice
  erythromycin 10
  ampicillin 17

kernicterus 11, 12

lactation (see breast feeding)
laryngitis 91
  adults 96
  children (croup)
    antibiotic use 94
    differential diagnosis 95
    epiglottitis 92
    laryngotomy 94
    laryngo-tracheitis 91
    steam 93
    steroids 95
lassa fever 50, 196
leptospirosis 197
Legionella pneumophila
  flu-like illness 196
  pneumonia 144

malaria 195
measles 49, 59, 66, 91, 103, 141, 154, 181, 183, 187
meningism 191, 201
methotrexate
  sulphonamides 16
metronidazole
  alcohol 16
  breast feeding 12
  contraceptive pill 7
  Giardia lamblia 172
  otitis media 71, 79
  pneumonia 154
  pregnancy 9
  sinusitis 86
  tonsillitis 53
    glandular fever 59
    quinsy 48
  warfarin 16
myalgic encephalomyelitis 192
myasthenia gravis
  aminoglycosides 16

Index

Mycoplasma pneumoniae
  flu-like illness 195
  otitis media 72
  pneumonia 141
  simple respiratory illness 104
  wheezy bronchitis 122, 127
myocarditis, acute 192

nalidixic acid
  neonates 13
  pregnancy 11
  shigella 171
  urinary infection 187
  warfarin 16
neomycin 13
neonates
  antibiotic use 13
nitrofurantoin
  elderly 14
  neonates 13
  pregnancy 11
  urinary infection 187

oesophageal ulcer
  antibiotic causation 14
otitis media 98
  antibiotic use 73
  auroscope use 65
  bacteria 71
  chronic 78
  flu-like illness 192
  PUO 182
  recurrent 70
  secretory 71, 72, 78
oxygen 165

paracetamol 37
parainfluenza viruses 51, 66, 91, 100, 121, 147, 193
parvovirus 183
patterns of illness 27, 100, 135, 190
penicillin
  allergy 1
  breast feeding 12
  contraceptive pill 7
  otitis media 74
  pneumonia 149
  pregnancy 9
  tonsillitis 57
pericarditis 192
pertussis 103, 110, 116, 154
  antibiotic uses 104, 110
  steroids 111
pharyngitis 42, 45, (see tonsillitis)

gonococcal 49
ulcers 49
pneumonia
  antibiotic use 149
  aspiration 148
  β-haemolytic streptococcus 148
  cardiac failure 138, 153
  Chlamydia psittaci 145
  Chlamydia trachomatis 148
  clinical diagnosis 135
  collapse (pulmonary) 154
  Coxiella burnetii 146
  flu-like illness 192, 194
  Gram negative bacteria 148
  Haemophilus influenzae 147
  home management 149
  illness course 152
  immunosuppression 148
  investigation 138, 140
  Legionella pneumophila 144
  lipoid 148
  measles 148, 154
  Mycoplasma pneumoniae 141
  'not pneumonia' 154
  pertussis 148, 154
  predominant pleuritic pain 155
  PUO 183
  Staphylococcus aureus 146
  Streptococcus pneumoniae 141
  tuberculosis 138, 148
  unresolved 153
  viral causes 147
poliomyelitis 195
  immunisation 4
pregnancy
  antibiotics and the contraceptive pill 7, 8
  antibiotic safety 8
pseudomembranous colitis 6
psittacosis (see *Chlamydia psittaci*)
PUO
  adults 199
  children 181
pyrexia 31
  delirium 34
  febrile apnoea (infants) 36
  febrile convulsions 31
  Reye's syndrome 37
  rigors 34
  symptomatic management 35

Q-fever (see *Coxiella burnetti*)
quinsy 48, 60

renal failure and antibiotics   15
  breast feeding   13
  elderly   14
respiratory syncytial virus   66, 91, 100,
    147, 159, 193
Reye's syndrome   37, 193
rhinitis
  allergic   84, 106, 115
  vasomotor   107
rhinoviruses   51, 66, 91, 100, 121, 147,
    193
ribavirin   153, 160, 203
rifampicin   7
rigors   34
roseolar infantum   183
rotavirus   66, 103, 169, 181
rubella   183

salmonella   170
  typhoid   196
scarlet fever   48
selective antibiotic use, principles   22
septicaemia   194
shigella   171
sinusitis   83, 115
  antibiotic use   88
  bacteria   86
  flu-like illness   192
  PUO   182
smoking   161, 162
  passive   114
sore throat   41
  inflamed   45 (see tonsillitis)
  non-inflamed   43
steam   93, 96, 102
steroids
  asthma   123, 129
  chronic obstructive airways
    disease   162
  croup   95
  pertussis   111
Staphylococcus aureus   71, 79, 87, 95,
    146, 166, 167, 173
Streptococcus pneumoniae   71, 86, 106,
    141, 160, 164
Streptococcus suis Type II, 198
swallowing
  oesophageal ulcer   14

teeth
  tetracycline staining   11, 13
temperature (see pyrexia)
tepid sponging   34, 38

tetracycline
  absorption   17
  allergy   5
  breast feeding   12
  chlorpropamide   16
  chronic obstructive airways
    disease   164
  contraceptive pill   7
  elderly   14
  neonates   13
  pneumonia   152
  pregnancy   11
  teeth staining   11, 13
  yersinia   172
theophylline
  erythromycin toxicity   15
tonsillitis   41
  antibiotic use   54
    prophylaxis   59
  bacteria and viruses   51
  diphtheria   49
  flu-like illness   191
  glandular fever   48, 58
  measles   49, 59
  PUO   183
  quinsy   48, 60
  scarlet fever   48
  tonsillectomy   60
toxoplasmosis   198
training
  the patient   26
  the doctor   27
trimethoprim (see co-trimoxazole)
  urinary infection   187
tuberculosis   115, 138, 148, 161
typhoid   196

urinary infection
  children   184, 187
  adults   194

vancomycin   6, 173
vomiting
  non-specific   169
  gastro-enteritis   169
    anti-vomiting drugs   178
    differential diagnosis   174

warfarin
  antibiotics   16
wheezy bronchitis (see asthma)
whooping cough (see pertussis)

yersinia   172

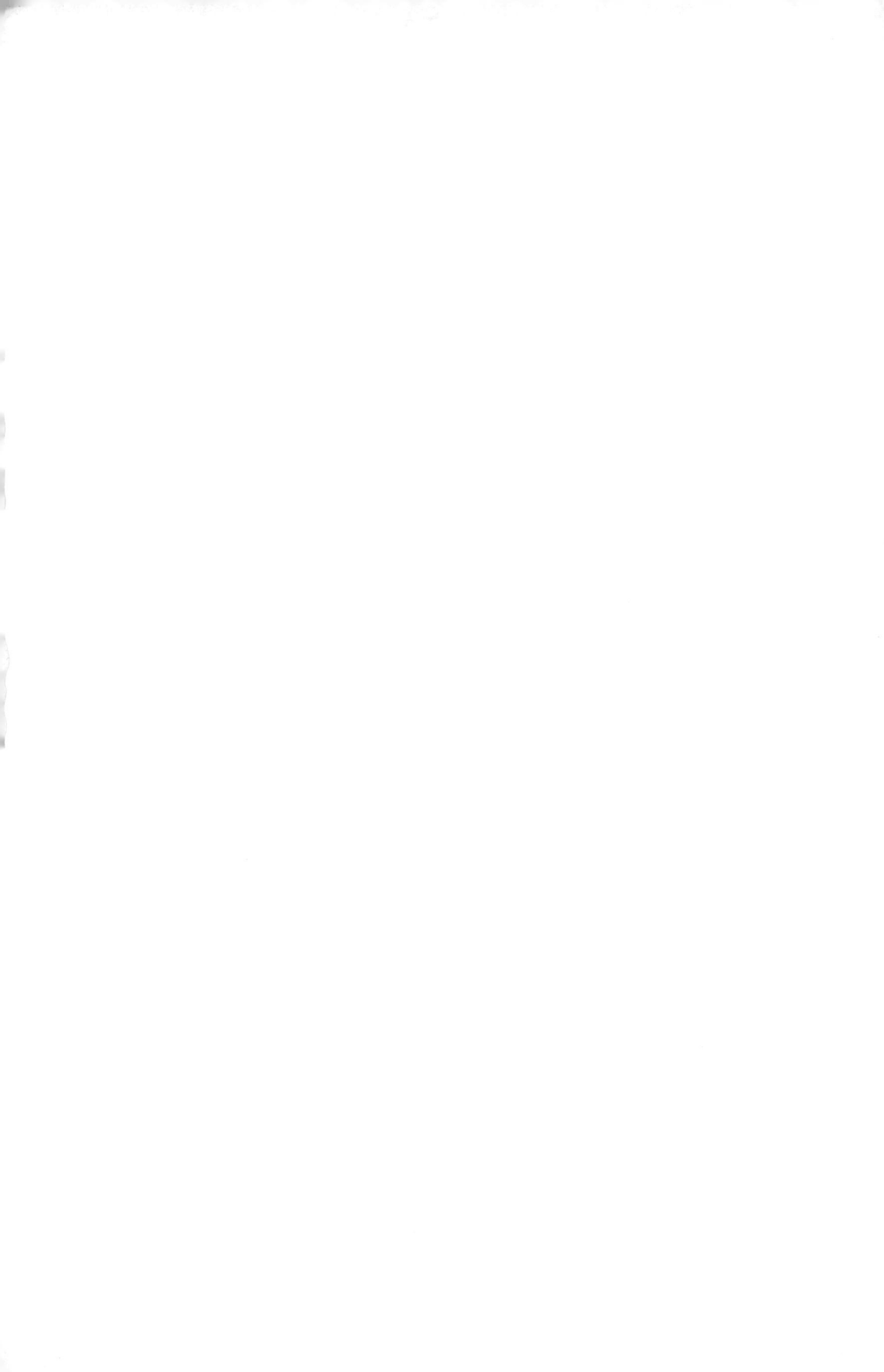

GPSR Compliance

The European Union's (EU) General Product Safety Regulation (GPSR) is a set of rules that requires consumer products to be safe and our obligations to ensure this.

If you have any concerns about our products, you can contact us on

ProductSafety@springernature.com

In case Publisher is established outside the EU, the EU authorized representative is:

Springer Nature Customer Service Center GmbH
Europaplatz 3
69115 Heidelberg, Germany